ENDOCRINE SURGERY

The HANDBOOKS of OPERATIVE SURGERY

THE STOMACH AND DUODENUM (5th ed.)

CLAUDE E. WELCH, M.D.
Visiting Surgeon, Massachusetts General Hospital
Clinical Professor of Surgery, Harvard Medical School

SURGICAL GYNECOLOGY (4th ed.)

J. P. GREENHILL, M.D. (Deceased)
Professor of Gynecology, Cook County Graduate School of Medicine
Senior Attending Obstetrician and Gynecologist, Michael Reese Hospital
Attending Gynecologist, Cook County Hospital

THE CHEST (4th ed.)

JULIAN JOHNSON, M.D., D.Sc. (Med.)
Professor of Surgery, School of Medicine, University of Pennsylvania

HORACE MACVAUGH, III, M.D.
Assistant Professor of Clinical Surgery, School of Medicine, University of Pennsylvania

JOHN A. WALDHAUSEN, M.D.
Professor of Surgery and Chairman, Department of Surgery,
Milton S. Hershey School of Medicine, Pennsylvania State University

THE BILIARY TRACT, PANCREAS AND SPLEEN (4th Ed.)

CHARLES B. PUESTOW, M.D.
Clinical Professor of Surgery, The Abraham Lincoln School of Medicine and
Graduate College, University of Illinois

SURGICAL UROLOGY (4th ed.)

R. H. FLOCKS, M.D.
Professor and Head, Department of Urology

DAVID CULP, M.D.
Professor of Urology, University of Iowa College of Medicine

THE HEAD AND NECK (3d Ed.)

ROBERT A. WISE, M.D.
Clinical Professor of Surgery

HARVEY W. BAKER, M.D.
Associate Clinical Professor of Surgery, University of Oregon Medical School

CARDIOVASCULAR SURGERY (2d ed.)

ORMAND C. JULIAN, M.D., PH.D.
Professor of Surgery

WILLIAM S. DYE, M.D.
Clinical Professor of Surgery

HUSHANG JAVID, M.D., PH.D.
Professor of Surgery

JAMES A. HUNTER, M.D.
Associate Professor of Surgery

HASSAN NAJAFI, M.D.
Associate Professor of Surgery, The Abraham Lincoln School of Medicine, University of Illinois

---

SURGERY OF THE BREAST

HARRY W. SOUTHWICK, M.D.
Clinical Professor of Surgery, The Abraham Lincoln School of Medicine, University of Illinois

DANELY P. SLAUGHTER, M.D. (Deceased)
Clinical Professor of Surgery, The Abraham Lincoln School of Medicine, University of Illinois

LOREN J. HUMPHREY, M.D.
Associate Professor of Surgery, Emory University School of Medicine

---

REPAIR OF HERNIAS

MARK M. RAVITCH, M.D.
Professor of Surgery, University of Pittsburgh School of Medicine, and Surgeon-in-Chief, Montefiore Hospital, Pittsburgh

---

SURGERY OF THE SMALL AND LARGE INTESTINE

HERBERT B. GREENLEE, M.D.
Chief of Surgery, Veterans Administration Hospital, Hines, Illinois
Professor of Surgery, Loyola University Stritch School of Medicine

---

ORTHOPAEDIC SURGERY

EDWARD L. COMPERE, M.D.
Chief of Orthopaedic Surgery, Medical Center Clinic and Hospital of El Monte, California
Edwin Warner Ryerson Professor and Chairman, Emeritus,
Department of Orthopaedic Surgery, Northwestern University

ENDOCRINE SURGERY

EDWARD PALOYAN, M.D.
Associate Chief of Staff for Research, Chief of Endocrine Surgery, Veterans Administration Hospital, Hines, Illinois, Professor of Surgery, Loyola University Stritch School of Medicine

A. M. LAWRENCE, M.D., PH.D.
Associate Chief of Staff for Education, Program Director, Endocrinology-Diabetes, Veterans Administration Hospital, Hines, Illinois; Professor of Medicine and Biochemistry, Loyola University Stritch School of Medicine

A HANDBOOK OF OPERATIVE SURGERY

ENDOCRINE SURGERY

by

EDWARD PALOYAN, M.D.

Associate Chief of Staff for Research, Chief of Endocrine Surgery, Veterans Administration Hospital, Hines, Illinois; Professor of Surgery, Loyola University Stritch School of Medicine, Maywood, Illinois

A. M. LAWRENCE, M.D., Ph.D.

Associate Chief of Staff for Education, Program Director, Endocrinology-Diabetes, Veterans Administration Hospital, Hines, Illinois; Professor of Medicine and Biochemistry, Loyola University Stritch School of Medicine, Maywood, Illinois

Illustrated by Diane Nelson

YEAR BOOK MEDICAL PUBLISHERS • INC.
35 EAST WACKER DRIVE • CHICAGO

Copyright © 1976 by Year Book Medical Publishers, Inc. All rights reserved. No part of this publication may be reproduced, stored in a retrieval system, or transmitted, in any form or by any means, electronic, mechanical, photocopying, recording, or otherwise, without prior written permission from the publisher. Printed in the United States of America.

Library of Congress Catalog Card Number: 75-40526

International Standard Book Number: 0-8151-6625-7

DEDICATED TO
OUR RESPECTIVE FAMILIES

And

GEORGE E. BLOCK, M.D.

ROBERT J. FREEARK, M.D.

HERBERT B. GREENLEE, M.D.

PAUL V. HARPER, M.D.

Preface

MEDICAL ENDOCRINOLOGY has been an established field for over 50 years. Endocrine pathology has been a discipline of special interest for a number of surgical pathologists in this decade, as shown by the publication of textbooks and monographs assigned to this field. In view of these developments it is surprising that endocrine surgery as a special interest has lagged in gaining recognition.

The principal reason that endocrine surgery has not loomed as a special area is undoubtedly the relatively small volume of cases and the distribution of those few cases among already established surgical specialties such as neurosurgery (pituitary), urology (adrenal), gynecology, head and neck and general surgery.

Surgical endocrinology, however, is fast emerging as a discrete discipline, as increasing numbers of surgeons choose to devote their clinical knowledge and scholarly pursuits to diseases of the endocrine system.

In addition to the intellectual challenge of an ever-changing base of knowledge and a fascinating spectrum of diseases, the trend toward specialization among surgeons and the rewarding interchange drawn from collaboration between the endocrine pathologist and medical endocrinologist have fostered an atmosphere in which the endocrine surgeon can often serve as an equal partner in the care and disposition of patients with endocrine and metabolic diseases.

Added to these developments is the effect of modern technologies for early detection of endocrine aberrations, often at a time when surgical management may effect a cure not previously attainable. Who would have dreamed in 1960 that 10 years later one might operate upon a patient with a thyroid gland appearing normal to physical examination and scan, and with normal basal thyrocalcitonin levels, and find medullary carcinoma? Today the only indication for such an operation may be family history or an abnormal or exaggerated rise in circulating thyrocalcitonin following either a calcium or a pentagastrin infusion. Earlier diagnosis of hyperfunctioning endocrine disease, because of new and remarkably sensitive assays, now allows surgical intervention before gross pathology and extensive morbidity develop. Today, for example, a bilateral adrenalectomy for Cushing's disease may reveal adrenals of normal size and weight and a cortex which appears normal to gross inspection.

It seems fair to designate surgical endocrinology as a discrete discipline. This development can only serve to provide a more refined and rational therapeutic approach to many endocrine diseases. Given the collaboration of surgeon, internist and pathologist in dealing with such clinical material, a new and sounder knowledge of the pathogenesis and the natural course of endocrine diseases will clearly be forthcoming.

Finally, as authors we would not feel comfortable if we did not make three specific acknowledgments: to Dr. Richard H. Egdahl, who is a source of inspiration, to Mr. Fred A. Rogers of Year Book Medical Publishers for his patience and to Mrs. Corrine Popelka, who suffered through the countless revisions with serenity and equanimity and was a constant reminder that this job had to be completed.

EDWARD PALOYAN
A. M. LAWRENCE

Table of Contents

Chapter	Page
List of Illustrations	15
1. Surgical Diseases of the Parathyroid Gland	18
Historical Perspective	18
Regulation of Calcium Homeostasis	20
Differential Diagnosis of Hypercalcemia	22
Anatomy of the Parathyroid Glands	24
Location of Normal-Sized Parathyroid Glands	28
Location of Enlarged Parathyroid Glands	32
Primary Hyperparathyroidism	34
Clinical Forms	34
Clinical Signs and Symptoms	38
Abnormal Chemistries	40
Bone and Joint Signs	42
Disorders Associated with Hyperparathyroidism	44
Diagnosis	47
Parathyroidectomy	49
Mobilization of Thyroid Gland and Identification of All Four Parathyroids	52
Extent of Excision	54
Closure	54
Routine Postoperative Care	56
The First 24 Hours	56
The Second 24 Hours	59
Results of Parathyroidectomy for Primary Hyperparathyroidism	59
Pathology	59

Table of Contents

Chapter	Page
Tests for Hypocalcemia	60
Management of Hypocalcemia	60
Long-Term Follow-up in Parathyroidectomy	62
Parathyroid Autotransplantation	63
Re-exploration after Parathyroidectomy	63
Localization of Aberrant or Overlooked Tumors	64
Renal (Secondary) Hyperparathyroidism	68
Pathology	68
Diagnosis and Indications for Parathyroidectomy	69
Parathyroidectomy for Renal Hyperparathyroidism	70
Management of Special Circumstances	72
2. The Thyroid Gland	78
Embryology	80
Ectopic Thyroid Tissue	82
Surgical Anatomy	84
Pathophysiology from the Surgical Viewpoint	86
Thyrotoxicosis	86
Toxic Adenoma	87
Thyroid Tumors	87
Nontoxic Diffuse and Multinodular Goiters	88
Thyroid Tumors	88
Clinical Evaluation	90
Needle Biopsy of Nodules	92
Aspiration Cytology	92
Thyroglossal Duct Anomalies	92
Indications for Thyroidectomy	93
Preoperative Management in Thyroidectomy	94
Exposure of the Thyroid	94
Excision of Thyroid Nodule	96
Thyroid Lobectomy	100
Total Thyroidectomy	102
Total Thyroidectomy with Neck Dissection	104
Bilateral Subtotal Thyroidectomy for Graves' Disease	114
Thyroglossal Duct Cyst Excision	118
Lingual Thyroid Excision	120

Chapter	Page
Complications in Thyroid Operations	120
Postoperative Management	125
Thyrotoxic States	125
Benign and Malignant Tumors	125
3. Islet Cell Tumors of the Pancreas	126
Historical Highlights	126
Physiology of the Pancreatic Islets	130
Histology of the Pancreatic Islets	131
Classification of Islet Cell Tumors	134
Ectopic Location of Islet Cell Tumors	136
Pathology of Islet Cell Tumors	136
Embryology of the Pancreas	138
Anatomy of the Pancreas	140
Operative Approaches to the Pancreas	144
Exposure of Body and Tail by Division of Gastrocolic Ligament	148
Exposure of Head and Uncinate Process	152
Biopsy of Islet Cell Tumors	154
Hypoglycemia	156
Insulinomas	158
Diagnosis	158
Localization	160
Treatment	162
Resection of Tumors in Body or Tail of the Pancreas	164
Enucleation of Tumors in Head of the Pancreas	172
Excision of Tumors within the Uncinate Process	176
Enucleation of Ectopic Tumors	178
Postoperative Management	184
Medical Treatment of Beta Cell Tumors	184
Extrapancreatic Neoplasms	185
Gastrinomas	186
History	186
Clinical Manifestations	186
Diagnosis	188
Location in the Pancreas	190

List of Illustrations

	Plate
Normal Parathyroid Function	1
Developmental Anatomy of Parathyroid Glands	2
Anatomic Relationships of Parathyroid Glands	3
Location of Superior Parathyroid Glands	4
Location of Inferior Parathyroid Glands	5
Location of Enlarged Parathyroid Glands	6
Clinical Forms of Hyperparathyroidism	7
Renal Calcareous Disease	8
Abnormal Chemistries in Patients with Hyperparathyroidism	9
Radiographic and Other Signs in Hyperparathyroidism	10
Disorders Associated with Primary Hyperparathyroidism	11
Parathyroidectomy	12
Tests for Hypocalcemia	13
Arteriography in Localization of Overlooked Tumor	14
Venous Catheterization in Localization of Overlooked Tumor	15
Embryology of the Thyroid Gland	16
Ectopic Thyroid Tissue	17
Surgical Anatomy of the Thyroid Gland	18
Exposure of the Thyroid Gland	19
Excision of a Thyroid Nodule	20
Thyroid Lobectomy	21
Total Thyroidectomy	22
Total Thyroidectomy with Neck Dissection	23
Bilateral Subtotal Thyroidectomy for Graves' Disease	24

List of Illustrations

Plate

Thyroglossal Duct Cyst Excision 25
Histology of the Pancreatic Islets 26
Location of Islet Cell Tumors 27
Ectopic Locations of Islet Cell Tumors 28
Embryology of the Pancreas 29
Anatomy of the Pancreas 30
Blood Supply and Lymphatic Drainage of the Pancreas 31
Operative Approaches to the Pancreas 32
Exposure of Body and Tail of Pancreas 33
Exposure of Head and Uncinate Process of Pancreas 34
Management of Islet Cell Tumors 35
Location of Insulinomas 36
Pancreatic Resection for Insulinoma 37
Resection for Tumors in Body or Tail of the Pancreas 38
Enucleation of Tumors in Head of the Pancreas 39
Enucleation of Intraduodenal Ectopic Tumor 40
Total Gastrectomy for Gastrinoma 41
Embryology of the Adrenal Gland 42
Anatomy of the Adrenal Gland 43
Adrenal and Extra-adrenal Locations of Pheochromocytomas . . . 44
Abdominal Transperitoneal Approach to Right Adrenal Gland . . . 45
Abdominal Transperitoneal Approach to Left Adrenal
  with Reflection of the Spleen 46
Abdominal Transperitoneal Approach to Left Adrenal
  with Elevation of the Pancreas 47
Posterior Thoracolumbar Approach to Adrenal Glands 48

ENDOCRINE SURGERY

CHAPTER 1

Surgical Diseases of the Parathyroid Gland

WHY DOES HYPERPARATHYROIDISM mesmerize so many clinicians, investigators and basic scientists with such diverse backgrounds and interests? Perhaps the answer lies in the realization that the diagnosis of hyperparathyroidism and the decision to correct the disease must still be made on clinical grounds, despite the increasing accessibility of accurate serum calcium and parathyroid hormone (PTH) measurements to all clinicians in North America. The ravages of hyperparathyroidism and the effects of hypercalcemia cut across the boundary lines of many specialties. Most general surgeons, as well as those specializing in endocrine and head and neck surgery, enjoy the challenge of a "neck exploration" and the uncertainties they must face.

In other words, hyperparathyroidism remains in the 1970s a clinical and pathologic entity that provides the internist with an opportunity to demonstrate diagnostic skills and clinical judgment, and gives the surgeon a chance to demonstrate technical skills and a knowledge of anatomy.

Historical Perspective

The rhinoceros from which the first anatomic description of a parathyroid was drawn by Sir Richard Owen is still on display in the British Museum in London.

Milestones in the History of Hyperparathyroidism

1852
Sir Richard Owen describes the parathyroid glands in an Indian rhinoceros.

1880
Sandstrom discovers the parathyroids in man and other mammalian species.

1891
Von Recklinghausen describes osteitis fibrosa cystica.

1904
Askanazy describes a parathyroid tumor in a patient with osteitis fibrosa cystica.

1908–1909
MacCallum and Voegtlin discover that selective parathyroidectomy produces hypocalcemia and tetany, and correct this by the administration of calcium intravenously.

1924
Berman, Collip and Hanson separately isolate potent parathyroid extracts capable of raising serum calcium levels.

1925
Felix Mandl performs the first successful excision of a parathyroid tumor in Vienna on a streetcar conductor named Albert.

1928
The first successful parathyroidectomy in the United States was performed by I. Y. Olch at Barnes Hospital in St. Louis.

1960s
Purification and characterization of parathyroid hormone by H. Rasmussen, among others. Development of immunoassays for parathormone by C. Arnaud, E. Reiss, J. Canterburry, J. Potts, G. Aurbach, S. Berson and R. Yalow, among others.

Regulation of Calcium Homeostasis

The level of serum calcium is the end product of many dynamic forces regulated principally by a variety of hormonal mechanisms. The remarkable constancy of serum calcium is one of the wonders of biologic homeostasis. The daily dietary calcium requirement is approximately 1 gm in healthy adults and 3-4 gm in growing children and pregnant women. Absorption of calcium from the gastrointestinal tract is mediated through the action of vitamin D metabolites. Vitamin D is obtained either through ultraviolet-stimulated conversion of skin ergosterol or through the ingestion of vitamin-D-containing foods such as fish oils or vitamin-D-supplemented products such as bread, milk, flours and butter.

VITAMIN D.—Vitamin D is converted in the liver to a more active form, 25-hydroxycholecalciferol, and this product is in turn converted in the kidney into what is currently believed to be the active vitamin D metabolite, 1,25-dihydroxycholecalciferol. This renal conversion may require PTH. The active metabolites of vitamin D are believed to promote the synthesis of a calcium carrier protein within the gastrointestinal mucosa cell and to facilitate the absorption of calcium.

PARATHYROID HORMONE.—This hormone is a single-chain polypeptide of approximately 83 amino acid residues having an estimated molecular weight of 8,500. Secretion of PTH is primarily related to lowering of the ionized serum calcium level. This hormone acts on bone and on kidney function. It is believed to stimulate osteocytic osteolysis acutely, with osteoclastic stimulation occurring in response to chronic hypersecretion of the hormone. Osteocytic osteolysis is the principal mechanism for rapid mobilization of calcium from bone. Parathyroid hormone acts upon the kidney to reduce the clearance of calcium and to promote phosphate diuresis. It also acts in concert with vitamin D to enhance gut absorption of calcium. Parathyroid hormone exerts its action on bone and kidney by stimulating adenyl cyclase with the formation of $3',5'$-cyclic adenosine monophosphate (AMP). Cyclic AMP, in turn, has been found to stimulate bone calcium resorption and release into the bloodstream. Studies have also indicated that PTH-induced renal excretion of phosphorus is preceded by augmented excretion of cyclic AMP in the urine.

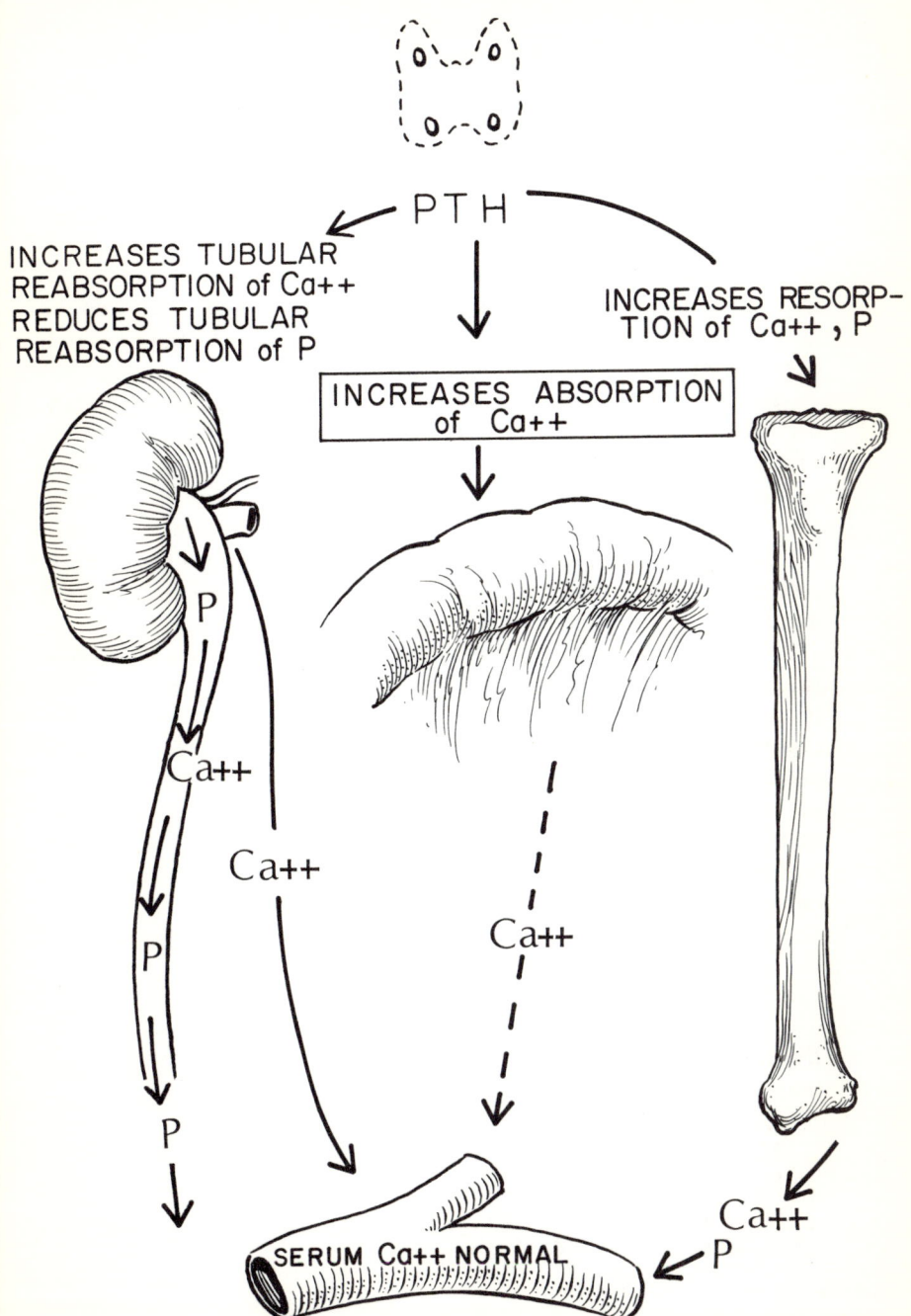

CALCITONIN. — In 1960 a new hormone, calcitonin, was discovered. This peptide is of thyroidal origin but stems from cells within the thyroid now believed to be of neural crest origin. Thyroid calcitonin acts to inhibit bone calcium resorption. Its clinical importance relates to C cell or medullary cancer of the thyroid, and its therapeutic use is in the treatment of severe osteoporosis and Paget's disease. Medullary thyroid cancer may produce large amounts of thyroid calcitonin, but because of counterregulatory influences hypocalcemia seldom develops. Absence of thyroid calcitonin, as may occur following total thyroidectomy, appears to have no discernible effect on calcium homeostasis in man.

INFLUENCE OF OTHER HORMONES. — Glucagon, the hyperglycemic, glycogenolytic principle secreted by the alpha cell of the islets of Langerhans (among other sites in the upper gut), may exert a regulatory influence on calcium balance by promoting renal excretion of calcium and by inducing a negative magnesium balance, which acts to interfere with the peripheral effects of PTH. There is also considerable evidence that the hypocalcemic effect of glucagon is mediated by the release of calcitonin.

Finally, some mention should be made of the probable role of the anabolic sex steroids, estrogens and androgens, as ameliorating influences in hyperparathyroidism. These hormones, by partially reversing the catabolic effects of PTH on bone matrix, can act to counter the hypercalcemia of hyperparathyroidism. Thus, it may be that the widespread use of birth control pills and the more frequent use of estrogens to alleviate the symptoms of the menopause will result in masking the peripheral signs of hyperparathyroidism caused by hypercalcemia.

Differential Diagnosis of Hypercalcemia

As hypercalcemia immediately raises the possibility of primary hyperparathyroidism, it is necessary to consider other diseases that may produce hypercalcemia, such as the following:
Sarcoidosis
Multiple myeloma
Lymphomas
Other neoplastic diseases
Vitamin D intoxication

Hyperthyroidism
Cushing's syndrome
Milk-alkali syndrome
Paget's disease
Mediastinal adenopathy will be seen in patients with sarcoidosis. A specific protein electrophoretic pattern is characteristic of multiple myeloma. Vitamin D intoxication is suspected by history and by the concomitant presence of hyperphosphatemia. Specific endocrinopathies, such as hyperthyroidism and Cushing's syndrome, should be obvious. Patients with visceral and other occult malignancies, which produce a PTH-like substance immunologically and, in all likelihood, biologically close to a native parathyroid hormone, pose the diagnostic challenge. Patients with primary hyperparathyroidism almost invariably demonstrate a mild hyperchloremic metabolic acidosis, whereas patients with hypercalcemia due to malignant production of PTH-like substance commonly have a mild metabolic alkalosis. Osteopenia or osteoporosis, frequently a feature of hyperparathyroidism, is usually absent in these neoplastic diseases.

Anatomy of the Parathyroid Glands

DEVELOPMENTAL ANATOMY. — The embryology of the parathyroids is of considerable interest to surgeons, who must, when operating on a patient with hyperparathyroidism, find all 4 glands. When the young surgeon despairs at failure to find one or both of the inferior parathyroids, the more experienced colleague will enjoy the amazement of onlookers if he draws a thymus from the superior mediastinum, incises it and produces a tan-colored, well-rounded parathyroid gland or tumor.

One of the salient developmental features that must be appreciated is that the superior parathyroids (IV) have a more consistent final anatomic location, perhaps because their downward and dorsal migration covers a shorter distance. However, they may be located deep within the thyroid parenchyma and be surrounded completely by its capsule. The further migration of the third pouch derivatives (parathyroid III and thymus) leads to a less consistent location of the inferior (III) parathyroid glands. The relationship of the inferior parathyroid to the thymus and the inferior poles of the thyroid does indeed vary considerably. These glands may be found completely embedded within the thyroid substance, in the thymic capsule or deep within the anterior mediastinum.

The location of these glands will be described in greater detail in a subsequent section (Plates 4–6).

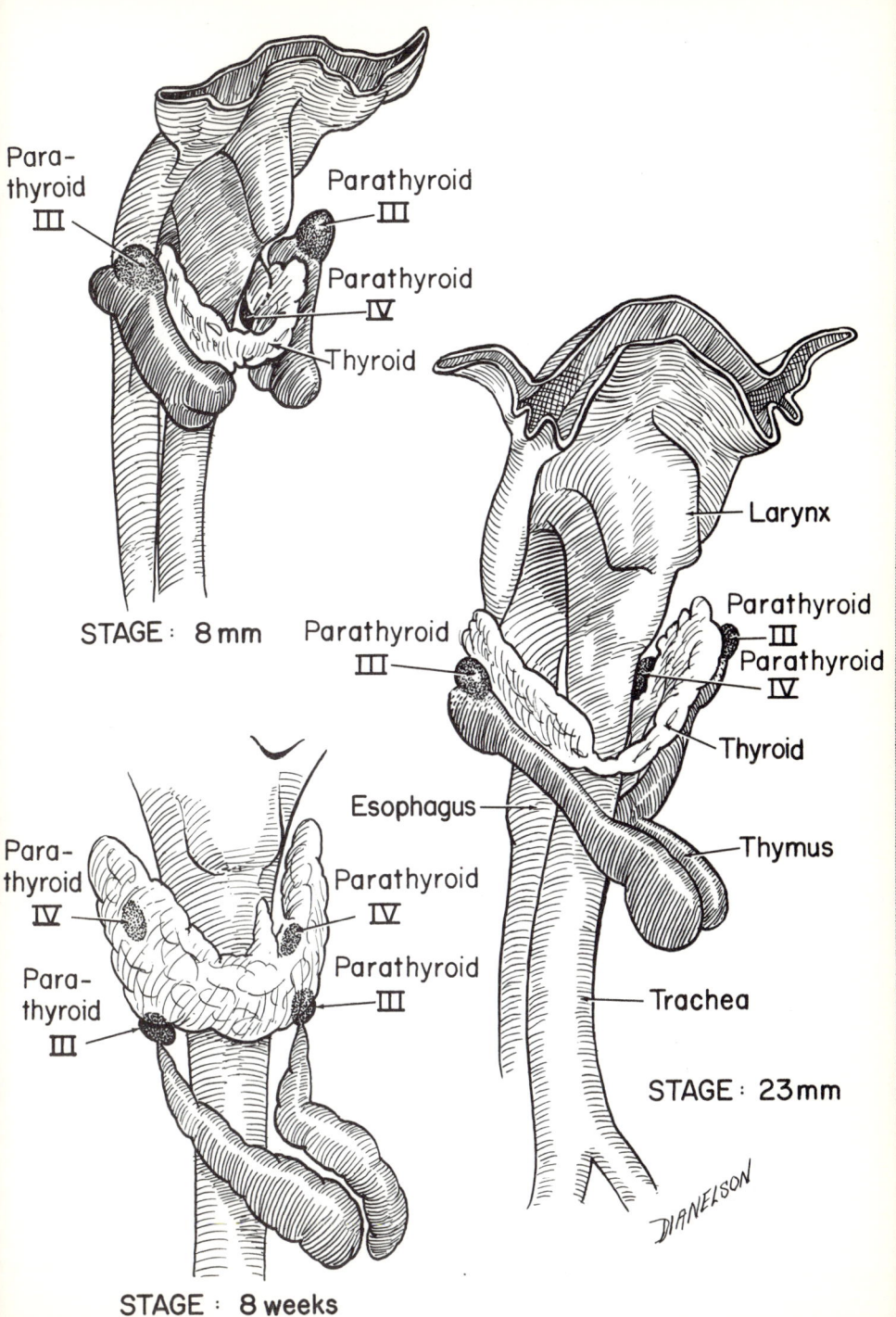

GROSS AND MICROSCOPIC APPEARANCE. — The gross characteristics of the parathyroid glands are learned best by dissection of fresh cadavers and in the surgical pathology laboratory, where the student takes note of their size, weight, color, contour, of the thin capsule and of the smooth and glistening cross-sectional surface. Each gland is a flattened, translucent, ovoid, soft, tan, smoothly encapsulated structure. Parathyroids weigh between 15 and 40 mg each. The combined weight of all 4 glands approximates 140 mg.

The rich blood supply to the parathyroids is derived from small branches of the superior and inferior thyroid arteries (Plate 3). The parathyroid veins join the superior middle and inferior thyroidal venous plexuses. Innervation of the parathyroids comes mainly from sympathetic fibers of the perivascular plexus. The lymphatic drainage extends to small peritracheal nodes, which in turn drain into the internal jugular lymph node chain.

Histologically the parathyroids are encapsulated by a thin collagenous wall, from which extend delicate fibrous septa, compartmentalizing the parenchyma. About one-half the cross-sectional area is made up of mature fat cells, while the remaining tissue is composed of vascular and parathyroid parenchyma with trabecular, alveolar or acinar arrangements. The main parenchymal cell is called the chief cell. The 2 others are the large polyhedral oxyphil cell, conspicuous by its bright eosinophilic cytoplasm, and the large vacuolated polyhedral parenchymal cell, commonly referred to as the water-clear cell. The chief cell is regarded as the basic parathyroid secretory cell, but there is no definite agreement as to the functional state of the water-clear and oxyphil cells. The amount of fat within the parathyroid varies with age. Little fat or fibrous tissue is evident in early childhood. During late childhood and adulthood more mature fat cells are deposited, until fat comprises approximately 50% of the adult gland. Oxyphil cells are absent in parathyroid tissue from young persons, but begin to appear by the prepuberal period and form clumps of 30–50 cells by middle adulthood.

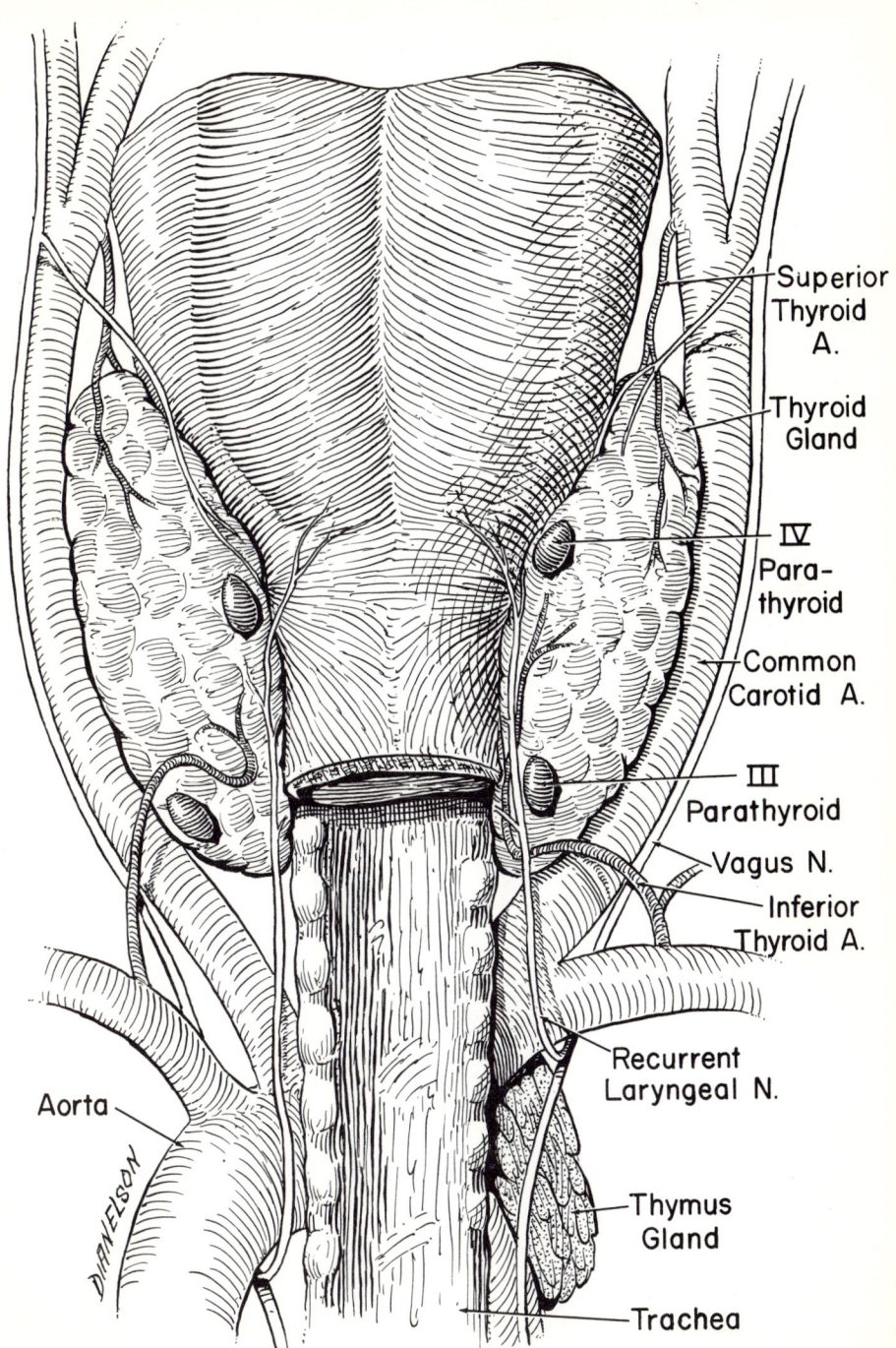

Location of Superior Parathyroid Glands

The superior parathyroids, which arise from the fourth pharyngeal pouch (IV) along with the thyroid anlage, descend during embryonic life, together with the thyroid, to their final position in the neck, close to the lateral posterior surface of the thyroid lobes. Since the superior parathyroids travel only a minimal distance during embryonic life, their final location is less varied than that of the inferior glands.

Characteristically the superior parathyroids are situated, one on each side, near the dorsal capsule of the thyroid gland at the level of the inferior border of the cricoid cartilage where the pharynx constricts to form the proximal esophagus (see Plate 3). From a lateral projection the superior parathyroid glands are most simply found by tracing the course of the recurrent nerve to its penetration of the cricothyroid membrane; it is at this location that the superior parathyroid glands are usually discovered. The stippled areas of Plate 4 depict the usual boundaries within which normal-sized superior parathyroids are ordinarily located. In less than 3% of subjects the superior gland may be buried within the lateral or superior lobe of the thyroid and can be discovered only after excision and sectioning of the ipsilateral thyroid lobe.

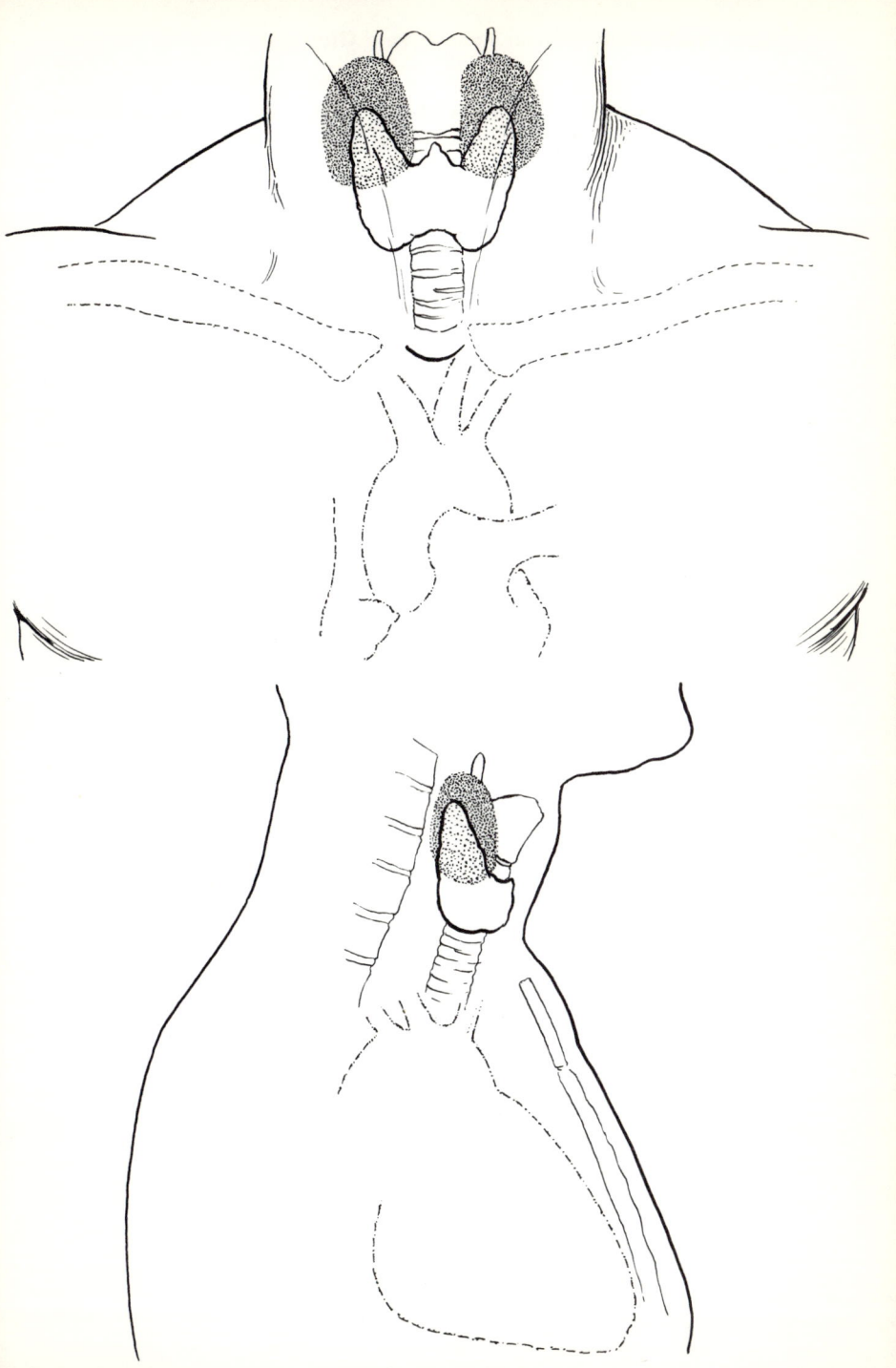

In contrast to superior parathyroid glands, normal-sized inferior parathyroid glands may be located over a wide area, presumably because the inferior glands, which arise from the third pharyngeal pouch (III), travel a longer distance along with the thymus. Usually the final position is close to the dorsal thyroid capsule at the level of the first tracheal ring, ventral to the tracheal margins and in close approximation to the inferior thyroid artery as it passes over and into the thyroid parenchyma. In 10–20% of individuals one or both inferior glands will be situated within the anterior mediastinum, frequently within the thymic capsule. These intrathymic parathyroids are usually located at the rostral end of the thymus, which extends cephalad up and out of the mediastinum, so that these glands can be reached through a cervical incision. Rarely a normal parathyroid gland may be located on the posterior surface of the thyroid between the trachea and esophagus, posterior to the esophagus, in the posterior superior mediastinum, within the vagus nerve close to the jugular foramen, deep within the thyroid substance or deep within the posterior mediastinum behind the carina.

PLATE 5

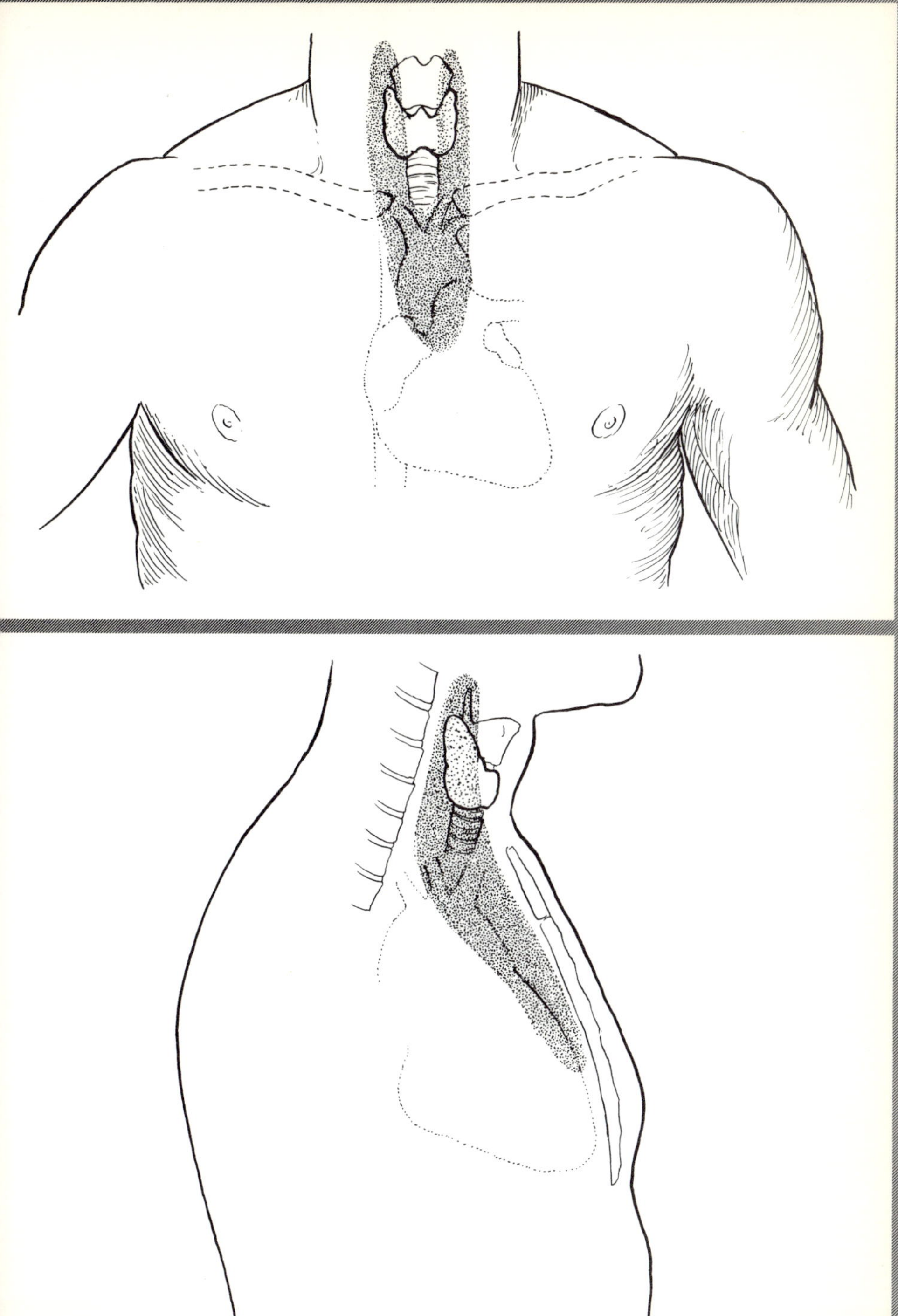

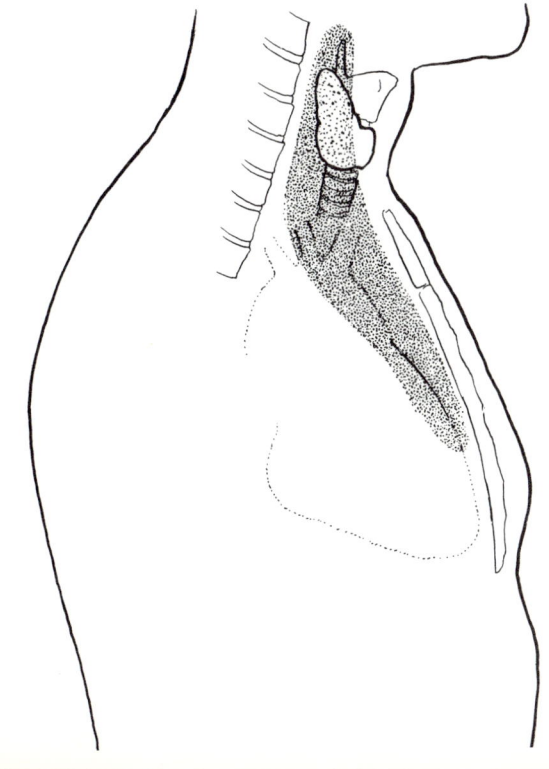

Abnormally enlarged parathyroid glands are much more likely to be ectopically located. It has been postulated that, because parathyroids lack fibrous attachment to the trachea or to other structures within the neck, they may be moved as they enlarge and bulge out of their original anatomic location. By the motions of swallowing and breathing they may be drawn to locations as high as well above the level of the thyroid cartilage or as low as the arch of the aorta, or between the aorta and the pulmonary artery in the anterior mediastinum or behind the carina in the posterior mediastinum. In any event, such glands usually have drawn their vascular pedicles from the original embryonic site. Localization of the ectopic glands is commonly facilitated by tracing these pedicles. Only in rare instances do aberrant glands derive their principal or collateral vascular supply from intrathoracic or other vessels.

Enlarged superior glands (IV) may migrate as high as the upper reaches of the thyroid cartilage and as far down as the arch of the aorta (A). They are often located in a retroesophageal position. However, they have *not* been described in the anterior mediastinum.

Enlarged inferior parathyroids (III) may be found both in the anterior and posterior mediastinum (B) and therefore can present a taxing challenge to the surgeon.

In chronic renal failure and secondary hyperparathyroidism, enlarged parathyroid glands are usually located within the boundaries described for normal parathyroid glands. This predilection for normal anatomic location is commonly ascribed to a general chronic inflammation within the neck that accompanies chronic renal disease and chronic dialysis.

PLATE 6

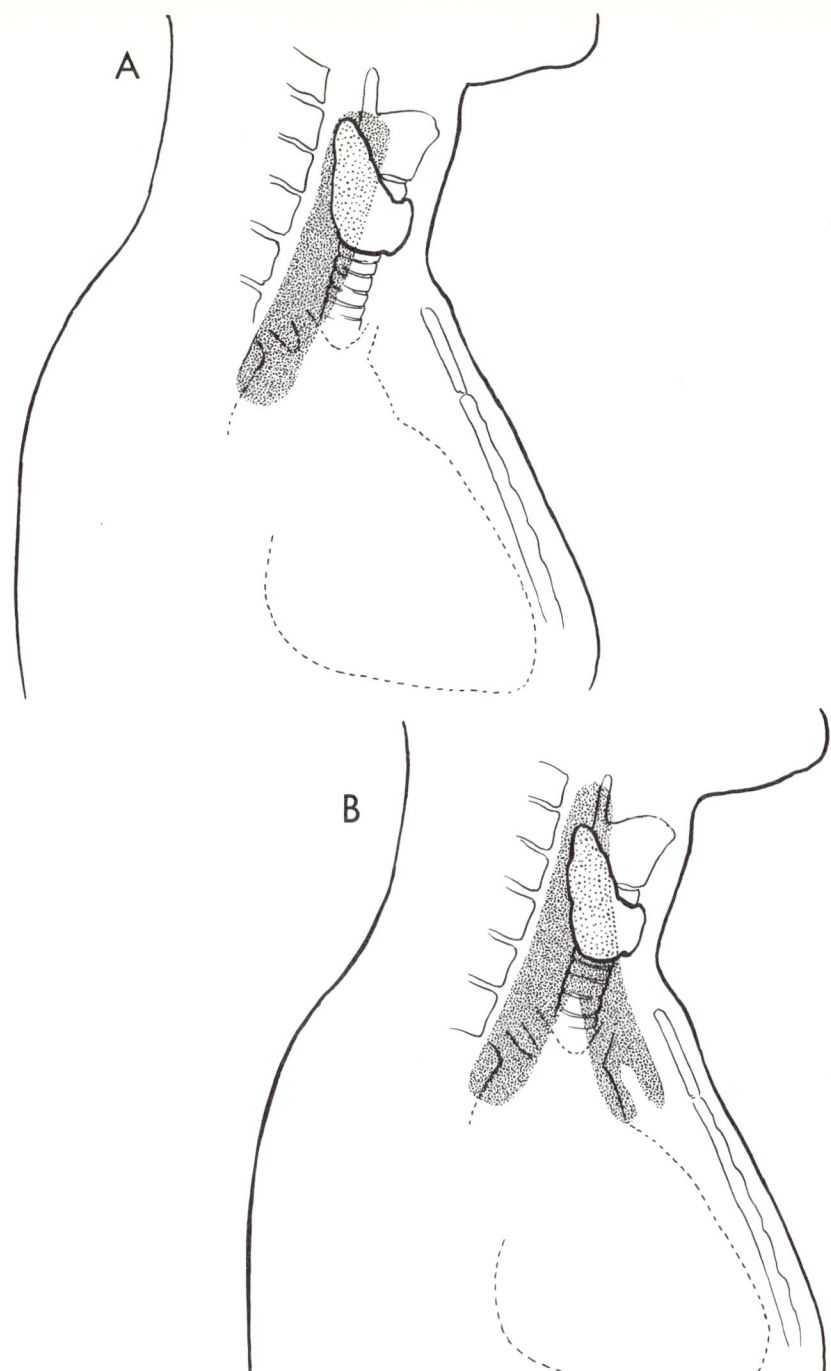

Primary Hyperparathyroidism

CLINICAL FORMS OF HYPERPARATHYROIDISM. — Patients with hyperparathyroidism may have:
1. Renal calcareous disease, either nephrocalcinosis and/or renal lithiasis
2. Hyperparathyroidism associated with definite bone involvement, osteopenia, subperiosteal resorption and osteitis fibrosa cystica
3. A combination of stone disease and bone involvement
4. Chemical hyperparathyroidism

Although these clinical forms overlap, a review of large series tends to reveal these fairly discrete clinical forms of hyperparathyroidism.

Patients with so-called chemical hyperparathyroidism are increasingly seen because of automated blood chemistry screening. Generally there is no detectable renal or bone involvement. However, they may have associated problems such as peptic ulcer disease or hypertension. On occasion such patients are noted to have spontaneous remission of the disease. Mild symptoms attributable to the hypercalcemia, such as fatigue, constipation, thirst and polyuria, may be present, however.

Probably because of earlier diagnosis of primary hyperparathyroidism, patients with severe bone disease are rarely seen today. When the skeleton is involved, such patients may have multiple large brown cystic tumors. This form of hyperparathyroidism seems more rapidly progressive once it is diagnosed; serum calcium levels are more markedly and persistently elevated. Generalized bone pain, myalgia and all the symptoms and signs attributable to hypercalcemia are usually present.

PLATE 7

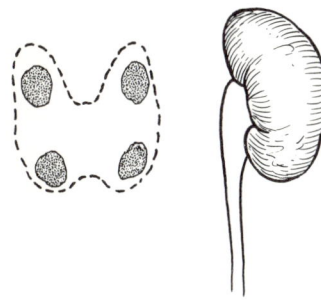

RENAL CALCAREOUS
DISEASE

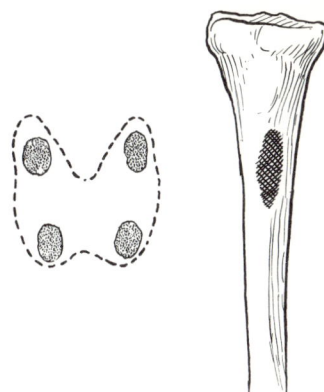

BONE CYSTS

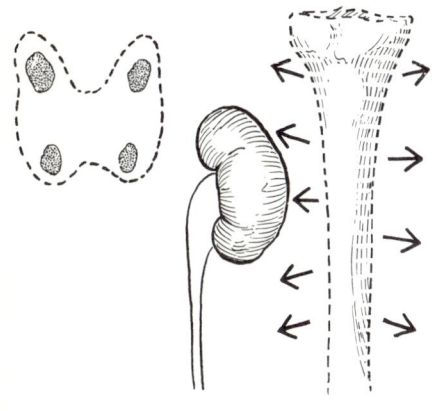

RENAL CALCAREOUS
DISEASE
AND OSTEOPOROSIS

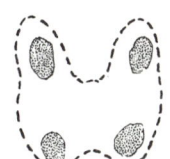

(Hypercalcemia,
Hypophosphatemia)

CHEMICAL DISEASE
WITH NO RENAL OR
BONE COMPLICATIONS

Patients with renal calcareous disease commonly have mild hypercalcemia, often with normal calcium levels interspersed with levels that are mildly elevated. This form of hyperparathyroidism appears to progress slowly, with the symptoms and signs secondary to metastatic calcification being more prominent than those accruing from hypercalcemia per se.

That some patients have stone formation and renal colic, whereas others have nephrocalcinosis with progressive damage to the renal parenchyma, remains an enigma (Plate 8). It may well be that there are 2 clinically distinct forms of hyperparathyroidism associated with renal calcareous disease and that we have not as yet learned to differentiate them.

In addition to identifiable clinical forms and their associated constellation of signs and symptoms, it is probable that, in the natural course of this disease, there are 3 pathologic stages:

1. An initial stage of potential reversibility, when elevated PTH levels can be suppressed with induced hypercalcemia, a state characterized by hyperplasia of 2 or more glands.

2. An intermediate stage, characterized by partial suppressibility of elevated PTH levels, with the presence of a mixture of hyperplasia and adenomas.

3. A late stage with 1 or more "adenomas" functionally autonomous and associated with atrophy of the remaining glands.

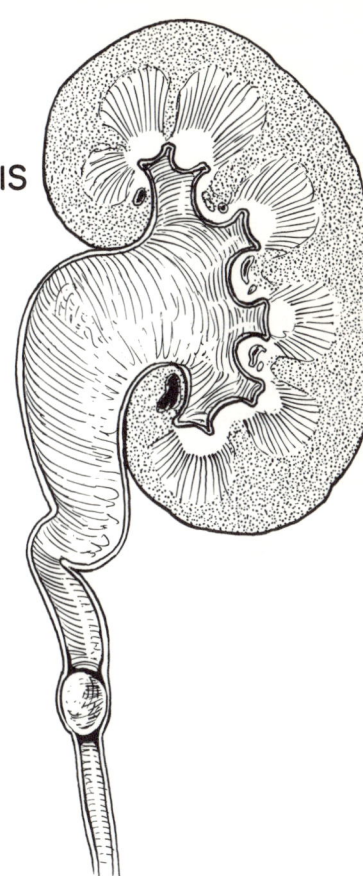
RENAL LITHIASIS

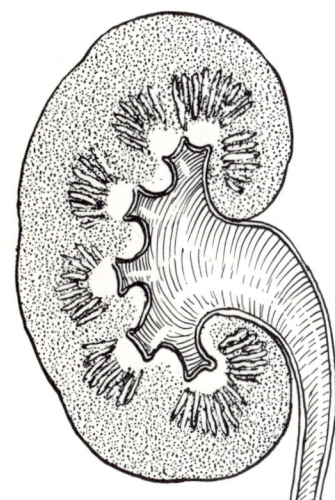
RENAL CALCINOSIS

Primary Hyperparathyroidism: Signs and Symptoms

CLINICAL SIGNS AND SYMPTOMS.—The symptoms and signs of primary hyperparathyroidism can be attributed to: (1) the unique catabolic effects of PTH on connective tissue ground substance, (2) hypercalcemia or (3) metastatic calcifications.

Excess PTH may induce the formation of renal stones. In addition, connective tissue ground substance is a primary target of the catabolic effects of PTH. The structural integrity of bone, the most specific connective tissue, may be particularly vulnerable in this regard. Patients may suffer from severe diffuse skeletal pain because of osteopenia and osteitis with bone cysts. Other effects of collagen degeneration include spontaneous and incisional hernias, hyperextensibility of joints, increased frequency of sprains, traumatic fractures from falls resulting from unstable joints, hemorrhoids and varicose veins. It is speculated that the higher incidence of peptic ulcer disease and pancreatitis in primary hyperparathyroidism may be due to a direct effect of excess PTH on these particular organs.

Hyperparathyroidism causes hypercalcemia, which in turn promotes metastatic calcification and diminished renal tubular concentrating ability, with polyuria, polydipsia and risk of dehydration. In addition, hypercalcemia impairs gastrointestinal motility and causes constipation, anorexia, nausea, and vomiting, which may further complicate dehydration. Generalized pruritus, ichthyosis, myalgia, arthralgias, muscle weakness and pseudogout may be seen as well. Hypercalcemia depresses central nervous system function, and psychiatric disorders, especially depression, are frequently present in the hypercalcemic patient. In addition to metastatic calcification in the kidneys, band keratitis may result from crystalline deposits of calcium phosphate salt in the limbus of the cornea. Hypercalcemia results in a shortened Q-T interval, enhances myocardial irritability, can cause increased digitalis sensitivity and may promote digitalis toxicity.

TABLE 1-1.—SIGNS AND SYMPTOMS OF PRIMARY HYPERPARATHYROIDISM

EFFECTS OF PTH EXCESS	EFFECTS OF HYPERCALCEMIA
Hypercalcemia, hypercalciuria Hypophosphatemia, hyperphosphaturia Hyperchloremia Glycosuria Renal stones (?)	Shortened Q-T interval (ECG) Myocardial irritability Digitalis sensitivity Renal stones, nephrocalcinosis Decreased renal tubular concentrating ability Polyuria, polydipsia and dehydration
Osteitis, bone pain Loss of lamina dura Brown tumors of bone Loose ligaments Spontaneous and incisional hernias Varicose veins, hemorrhoids Peptic ulcer disease (?) Pancreatitis (?)	Myalgias, muscular weakness Arthralgias, pseudogout Gastric hypersecretion Nausea, anorexia, constipation Pancreatitis CNS depression, psychiatric disorders Band keratitis

ABNORMAL CHEMISTRIES. — In hyperparathyroidism serum calcium levels are almost invariably raised. Parathyroid hormone promotes the resorption of bone salt and the gastrointestinal absorption of calcium and hence produces hypercalcemia, which results in the excretion of calcium by the kidney. Rarely patients with this disease may be eucalcemic. Factors that may promote lowering of the serum calcium level include vitamin D deficiency, estrogen administration, progressive renal insufficiency and possibly compensatory hypersecretion of such calcium-lowering hormones as thyrocalcitonin, glucagon and others.

Hypophosphatemia in the adult is due to PTH excess, renal tubular phosphate leak or dietary deficiency, such as may be seen in patients on long-term parenteral nutrition. Parathyroid hormone lowers the serum phosphate by inducing a phosphate diuresis, secondary to partial inhibition of renal tubular phosphate reabsorption. Patients with hyperparathyroidism who consume a diet rich in inorganic phosphates may not demonstrate hypophosphatemia.

For reasons not entirely understood, the serum uric acid is frequently elevated in hyperparathyroidism. A mild hyperchloremic metabolic acidosis is characteristic of primary hyperparathyroidism, and helps to distinguish the hypercalcemia of certain neoplasms from that due to excess PTH secretion. Results of 24-hour urinary calcium determinations may be above normal if the patient's serum calcium level is chronically raised above 12 mg/100 ml. In patients with hyperparathyroidism who have mild degrees of hypercalcemia and normal or raised phosphate clearance, the infusion of calcium (10 mg/kg) will fail to suppress phosphate clearance by more than 40%, as will occur in normal subjects.

Sensitive immunoassays for PTH may detect unequivocal elevations in peripheral blood, but on occasion this may only be detected in venous effluent draining the hyperplastic or adenomatous parathyroid tissue. Parathyroid hormone assay of selective venous catheterization sampling and arteriography may be needed to localize pathologic tissue.

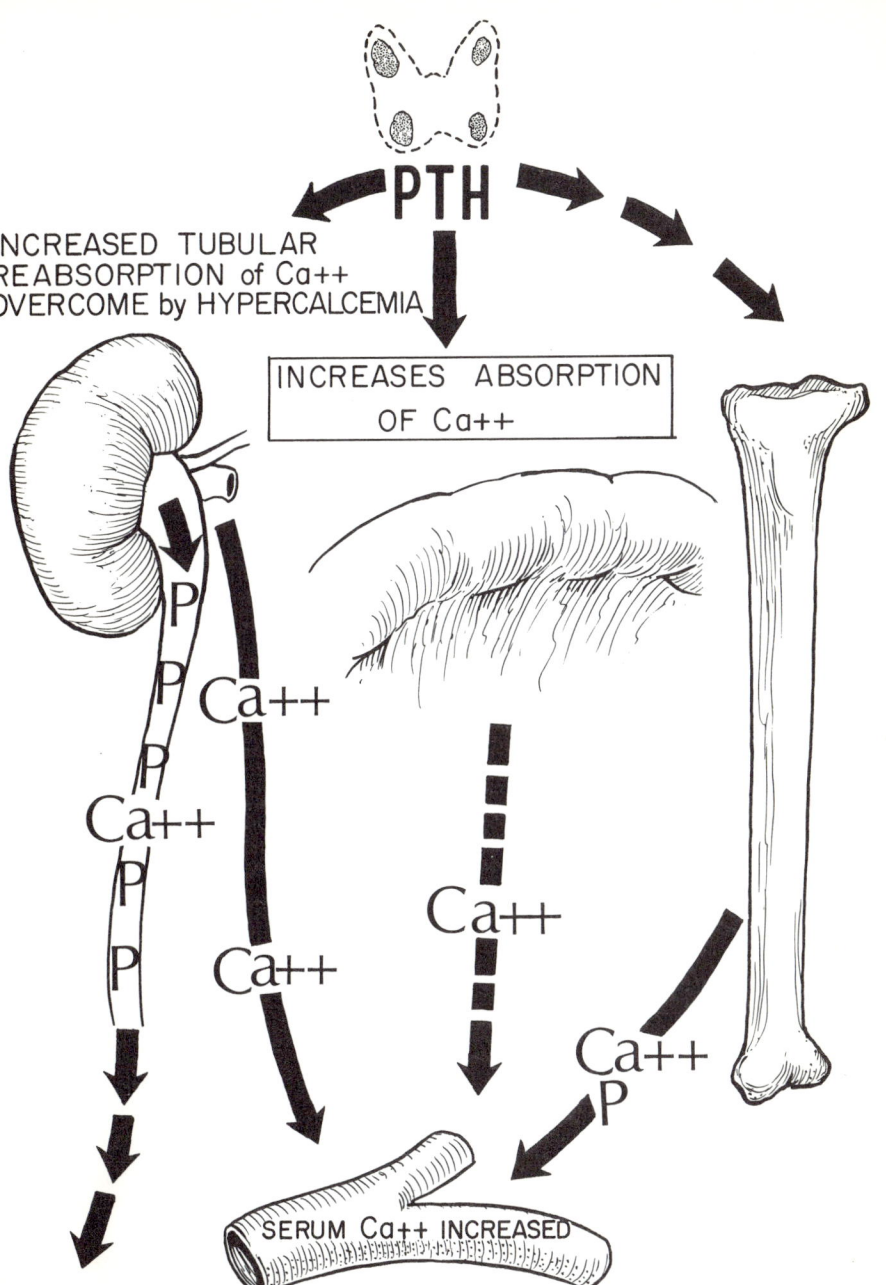

Hyperparathyroidism: Bone and Joint Signs

Signs that are typical of hyperparathyroidism include bone pain **(A)** which resolves completely within 48 hours after corrective parathyroid resection; hyperextensibility of joints secondary to catabolic loss of collagen **(B)**; decrease in height due to osteopenia of the vertebral column **(C)**; bone cysts **(D)**; periarticular metastatic soft-tissue calcifications **(E)**, primarily in secondary hyperparathyroidism; subperiosteal bone resorption **(F)**; loss of lamina dura **(G)**; remineralization of lamina dura following parathyroid resection **(H)**; and salt-and-pepper demineralization of the calvarium **(I)**.

The classic bone lesions of primary hyperparathyroidism are rarely seen in the population of patients with hyperparathyroidism today. Increased quantities of available dietary calcium, the stimulation of intestinal calcium absorption by added vitamin D in the American diet and the consumption of milk, which contains lactose, the calcium absorption-promoting disaccharide, all may act to retard PTH-induced negative calcium balance.

The classic skeletal lesions, infrequently seen today, include cystic brown tumors, demineralization of the calvarium (salt-and-pepper appearance), severe generalized osteopenia with shortened stature because of collapsed vertebrae and the "rugger-jersey" appearance of the vertebral column due to prominence of vertebral body end-plates, and periarticular metastatic calcification. The 2 last-named findings are peculiar to secondary (renal) hyperparathyroidism. Milder degrees of osteopenia may be detected by bone density measurements, and mild subperiosteal resorption of the phalanges of the hands may only be apparent in fine-detail industrial x-ray films used for such studies. Dental x-rays may reveal resorption of the lamina dura. Cervical angiography may help to delineate the exact site of enlarged glands. It may also be of invaluable assistance in localizing mediastinal tumors, especially after failure to discover the pathologic tissue at the first neck exploration.

PLATE 10

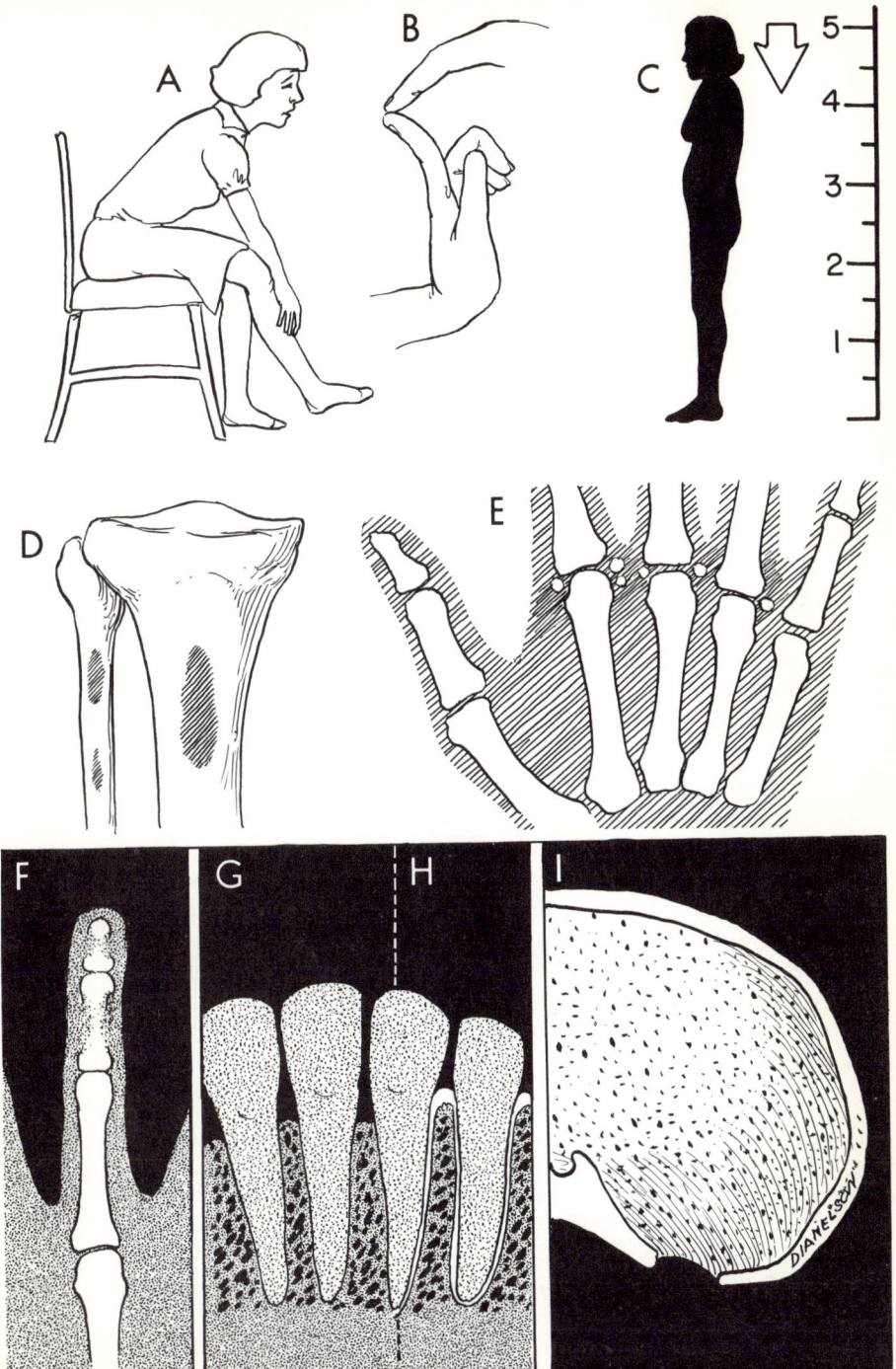

Disorders Associated with Primary Hyperparathyroidism

At this stage of our understanding of endocrine pathophysiology, hyperparathyroidism appears as the sole endocrinopathy in most instances. However, many patients have associated disorders that may well represent endocrine aberrations, and a few have outright endocrine tumors. These associations raise the possibility of etiologic relationships.

The incidence of hyperparathyroidism, which is 1 in 800 asymptomatic subjects undergoing routine physical examinations, is much higher in certain populations, such as patients with hypertension, peptic ulcer, chronic pancreatitis, pseudogout and thyroid tumors. Although a variety of hypotheses has been advanced to explain these associations, none is on a firm basis.

HYPERTENSION. — Hypertensive patients represent a heterogeneous population. The association of hypertension and hyperparathyroidism is partially explained by:

1. Hypertension caused by the multiple endocrine adenoma syndrome. For example, patients with Sipple's syndrome harbor bilateral pheochromocytomas as well as parathyroid tumors and medullary thyroid cancers. Patients with Cushing's syndrome and primary aldosteronism may also have hyperparathyroidism.

2. Hypertension treated by thiazide diuretics. Thiazide diuretics produce transient hypercalcemia and hypophosphatemia in most patients; prolonged administration of these agents has produced parathyroid hyperplasia in dogs and has been associated with hyperparathyroidism in some patients.

3. Hypertension may be the result of renal functional impairment caused by hyperparathyroidism, especially in patients with nephrocalcinosis.

In general, the correction of hyperparathyroidism may tend to facilitate the management of hypertension.

MULTIPLE ENDOCRINE TUMORS. — Patients with endocrine tumors have a propensity to develop other endocrine tumors; genetic predisposition may exist. There is no accepted explanation for the clinical varieties of these tumors.

THYROID TUMORS. — The incidence of thyroid nodules in hyperparathyroidism may be as high as 7%. A number of these may be medullary cancers. The development of hyperparathyroidism in a

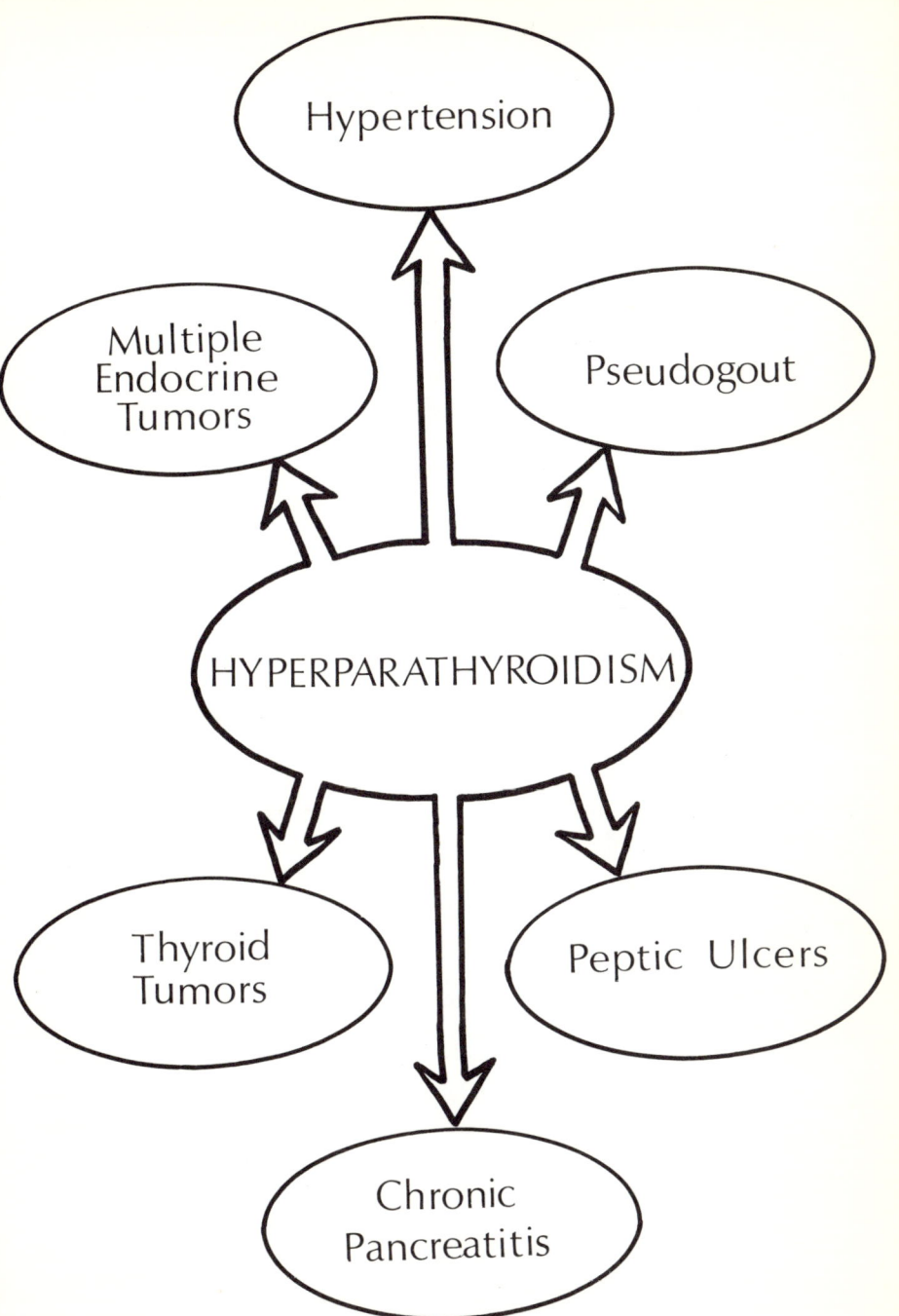

patient with calcitonin-secreting medullary cancer of the thyroid is plausible. There is no plausible rationale for the high incidence of other varieties of thyroid tumors in these patients.

CHRONIC PANCREATITIS.—Chronic pancreatitis, alcoholic or idiopathic, with its attendant malabsorption, may marginally pose a threat to optimal calcium absorption, thereby initiating chronic stimulation of the parathyroids with eventual development of parathyroid hyperplasia or adenoma formation. Further, it has been shown that hyperglucagonemia may be present in acute, and in many instances of subacute and chronic, pancreatitis. Glucagon also causes lowering of the serum calcium level, perhaps by stimulating the release of thyroid calcitonin. The sustained reduction of serum calcium in chronic pancreatitis may well be compensated by PTH hypersecretion and may set the stage for the development of hyperparathyroidism.

PEPTIC ULCERS.—Although the exact incidence of peptic ulcer in the general population is still uncertain, being on the order of 10%, an increased incidence of this disease is generally accepted in series of patients with primary hyperparathyroidism. The basis for this may be related both to hypercalcemia and to increased levels of circulating PTH. The former promotes increased gastric hydrochloric acid production; the latter may seriously compromise connective tissue healing and support. The heightened incidence of bleeding peptic ulcer in primary hyperparathyroidism is noteworthy in this regard.

PSEUDOGOUT.—The incidence of hyperparathyroidism in pseudogout has been reported to be as high as 30%. Correction of the disease does not relieve or ameliorate the symptoms of pseudogout.

CONCLUSIONS.—Large segments of our population are screened periodically for hypercalcemia by automated calcium and phosphorus determinations. Particular attention should be directed to the detection of hyperparathyroidism in the groups of patients just discussed, with determinations of serum calcium, phosphorus and PTH.

DIAGNOSIS AND INDICATIONS FOR PARATHYROIDECTOMY

The diagnosis of hyperparathyroidism can be made with relative ease in the majority of patients. For example, the combination of significant hypercalcemia, hypophosphatemia and hyperchloremia, documented over a period of several months, with no hint of an occult ectopic PTH-secreting tumor, constitutes sufficient grounds for proceeding with a parathyroidectomy.

The following is a list of diagnostic tests and procedures available to the clinician either locally, by mail or in a nearby university medical facility:

> Serum calcium, phosphate and chloride
> Serum PTH
> Renal clearance of phosphate
> Suppressibility of phosphate clearance
> 24-hour urine calcium
> Lamina dura x-ray
> X-rays of long bones, hands, clavicles, calvarium
> Fine-detail x-ray of hands (industrial film)
> Bone density measurement
> Bone biopsy
> Sampling of neck and thyroid veins for PTH
> Cervical and thyroid cervical angiography
> ^{75}Selenomethionine scanning
> Thermography

Documentation of elevated circulating PTH is desirable.

If the hypophosphatemia is equivocal, a high phosphate clearance or reduced tubular reabsorption of phosphate should be documented.

A more sensitive indication of parathyroid hyperplasia or adenoma is the demonstration of autonomy by the failure of intravenously induced hypercalcemia to suppress circulating PTH or phosphate clearance. The absence of a significant (>40%) fall in phosphate clearance (compared to baseline values) after calcium infusion is indicative of parathyroid autonomy and hyperparathyroidism. Some patients with renal impairment may not have any significant hypophosphatemia or increase in phosphate clearance.

Patients with renal calcareous disease and mild or equivocal hypercalcemia present the greatest diagnostic challenge. If the stone disease is caused by hyperparathyroidism, parathyroidectomy is usually effective in arresting its progression. However, if it is caused by idiopathic hypercalciuria, which features hypophosphatemia and occasionally mild hypercalcemia, parathyroidectomy will be futile. The problem is further compounded by the fact that both in idiopathic hypercalciuria and in this form of hyperparathyroidism the parathyroid glands may be moderately hyperplastic, and therefore even examination of the tissue may not clearly establish the diagnosis. An elevated circulating PTH is the best differential criterion if renal function is normal. The positive response of the patient to parathyroidectomy, in terms of the course of the stone disease, is the most important confirmatory evidence in favor of hyperparathyroidism.

In the chemical form of hyperparathyroidism, there is general agreement that parathyroidectomy is indicated by virtue of the significant hypercalcemia. The coexistence of hypertension or peptic ulcer strengthens the indications. In our laboratory, where the mean serum calcium level is 9.5 ± 0.3, any value of 11 and above repeated on several occasions over a period of 12 months is considered significant hypercalcemia.

Patients with the mild chemical form of the disease, with borderline hypercalcemia and no complications of hyperparathyroidism or associated syndromes, present problems created by the introduction of automation in the determination of serum calcium, which sifts these patients from the population at large.

No one knows how many of these patients have or will have the full clinical picture of hyperparathyroidism and how many will revert to normocalcemia. Do many patients become transiently hyperparathyroid in periods of stress to calcium metabolism or during periods of reversible renal impairment? There is general agreement that one should not rush in with parathyroidectomy in this group. The only controversial point is where one draws the line between significant hypercalcemia (presumably irreversible and requiring correction by parathyroidectomy) and mild (reversible?) hypercalcemia.

Patients with severe bone disease are rarely encountered these days. In the absence of neoplastic bone disease, the diagnosis of hyperparathyroidism is easily established in such patients. The indications for parathyroidectomy are clear.

In conclusion, once the diagnosis of hyperparathyroidism is made, and especially if complications and associated syndromes exist, parathyroidectomy is indicated. However, if a patient has only the mild chemical form, one can afford a period of observation to determine the course of the disease before reaching a decision.

Parathyroidectomy

Preoperative measures include assessment of vocal cord function and adequate hydration in patients scheduled for parathyroidectomy. Hypercalcemia causes the patient to pass a diluted urine; if fluid intake is not adequate, a serious degree of dehydration can result, which may in turn promote a hypercoagulable state. Since patients with hyperparathyroidism probably have an increased incidence of duodenal ulcer, with a propensity for active bleeding, it is wise that they be covered pre- and postoperatively with antacid therapy. Finally, when it seems warranted, patients and their families should be told that more than the usual psychologic distress may be encountered in the immediate postoperative period, a problem associated with a rapid readjustment of the serum calcium level toward normal. This usually takes the form of depression and is self-limiting within a few days postoperatively.

In general, upper respiratory infections contraindicate major operations, especially when general endotracheal anesthesia is required. This dictum is especially true in cervical operations such as parathyroidectomy that result in postoperative laryngeal and tracheal edema. An intercurrent upper respiratory infection would pose a serious threat of immediate postoperative laryngeal edema and airway obstruction.

ANESTHESIA.—The choice of the anesthetic agent depends in part upon the anesthesiologist. However, preoperative administration of opiates must be avoided; these trigger spasm of the sphincter of Oddi and predispose to pancreatitis in patients with hyperparathyroidism. Tracheal intubation is highly desirable. Placing of an esophageal stethoscope must be avoided, as such instrumentation interferes with neck dissections and increases the likelihood of trauma to laryngeal structures.

Local anesthesia may be dangerous in that inadvertent paralysis

[Technic of parathyroidectomy *on page 50.*]

of the vocal cords and airway obstruction may result from the diffusion of the local anesthetic to the recurrent laryngeal nerves or the vagal trunks from which they originate.

INSTRUMENTS.—Parathyroidectomy does not call for special instruments. Since the operation may involve the manipulation and dissection of fine vessels, which are small and delicate structures, fine-pointed instruments such as "baby" right-angle clamps and tenotomy scissors are useful.

POSITIONING.—Symmetry in positioning the head and neck helps to achieve a cosmetically symmetrical scar. A 30-degree elevation of the thorax **(A)** permits a drier field, since venous engorgement is thereby minimized.

INCISION AND DEVELOPMENT OF SKIN FLAPS.—A low curvilinear transverse cervical incision **(B)**, about 1.5 cm above the clavicles and 10–14 cm long, is used. Circumference and length of the neck as well as location of the thyroid determine the length of the incision. For cosmetic reasons the incision should seldom be made higher than 2 cm above the clavicle. The incision must be well planned and executed. By imprinting the skin at the desired level with a 00 suture the exact location for the incision can be "drawn." This is accomplished by having the assistant hold the center of the suture with a hemostat and place its tip at the center of the neck at an appropriate level above the manubrial notch, while the surgeon holds the 2 ends and presses this suture on the skin in the location he plans to make the incision. Finally, with a needle impregnated with methylene blue, pinpoint puncture marks are made on either side of the imprinted incision line; a ruler may be used to assure that the eventual incision will be symmetrical. These marks will be visible at the conclusion of the operation and will permit an accurate approximation of the skin edges.

The skin incision is made down to the platysma. The wound edges are protected with moist laparotomy pads from this point on.

The platysma is then incised transversely and flaps are developed up to the notch of the thyroid cartilage and down to the clavicles. Absolute hemostasis is essential.

The strap muscles are separated in the midline **(C)** and retracted laterally. An alternative approach, in patients with a short and

[Parathyroidectomy *continued on page 52.*]

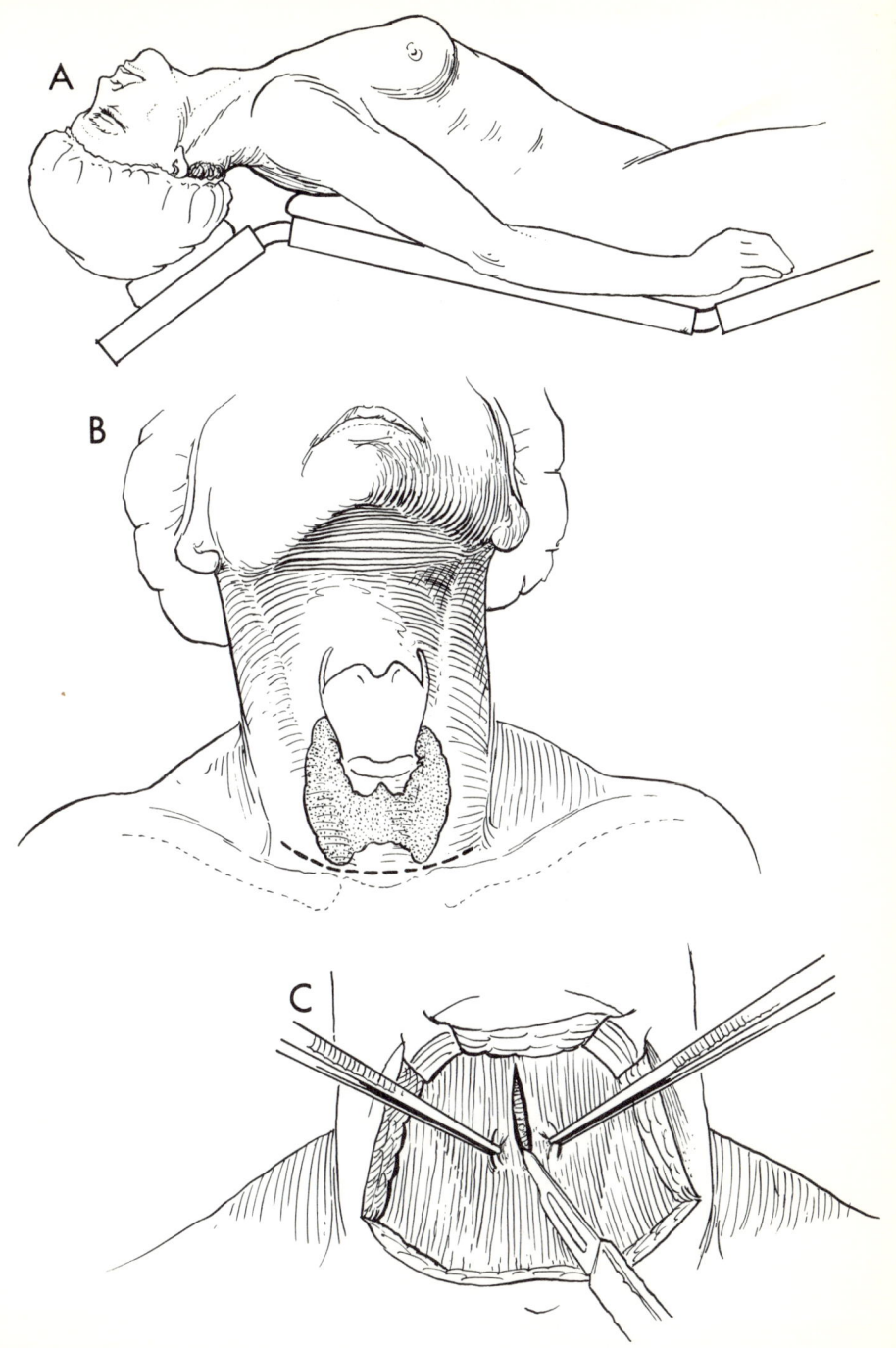

broad neck, is to transect these muscles to achieve adequate exposure.

MOBILIZATION OF THYROID GLAND AND IDENTIFICATION OF PARATHYROIDS.—All 4 parathyroid glands should be identified before a decision is made as to which glands will be resected. Both lobes of the thyroid are mobilized **(D** and **E)** by dividing the middle thyroid veins. A heavy suture is used to transfix the midportion of the thyroid and to facilitate further retraction and dissection. After identification of all 4 glands, specimens are removed **(F)** for histologic evaluation.

If all 4 glands cannot be visualized, the dissection proceeds further by dividing the superior pole vessels. The recurrent nerve is identified and traced to the point where it penetrates the cricothyroid membrane; as a rule, the superior parathyroid gland is situated near that point.

To expose a missing inferior gland, the inferior thyroid vessels are divided and the ipsilateral thymus dissected; as much of it as possible is excised. It may contain the missing gland.

The retroesophageal area is another common site of an aberrant gland. A thorough search will include the anterior and posterior superior mediastinum. All vascular pedicles arising from thyroid vessels should be traced, as they may lead to a missing parathyroid gland.

Finally, a missing gland may be located within the substance of the thyroid; before the operation is concluded the thyroid lobe on that side must be excised and examined.

If the search described fails to disclose a missing gland, a thorough reexamination is made of the sites that have been dissected, and an appropriate amount of parathyroid tissue is excised. All vascular pedicles arising from the thyroid vessels and leading to the mediastinum are ligated and divided, and the operation concluded. A formal sternum-splitting mediastinal exploration is not carried out at this time. On occasion and despite failure to discover and resect the offending tissue, the patient becomes euparathyroid following the neck dissection described. In all likelihood this is because of the disruption of the vascular supply to the hyperfunctioning parathyroid tissue.

[Parathyroidectomy *continued on page 54.*]

PLATE 12

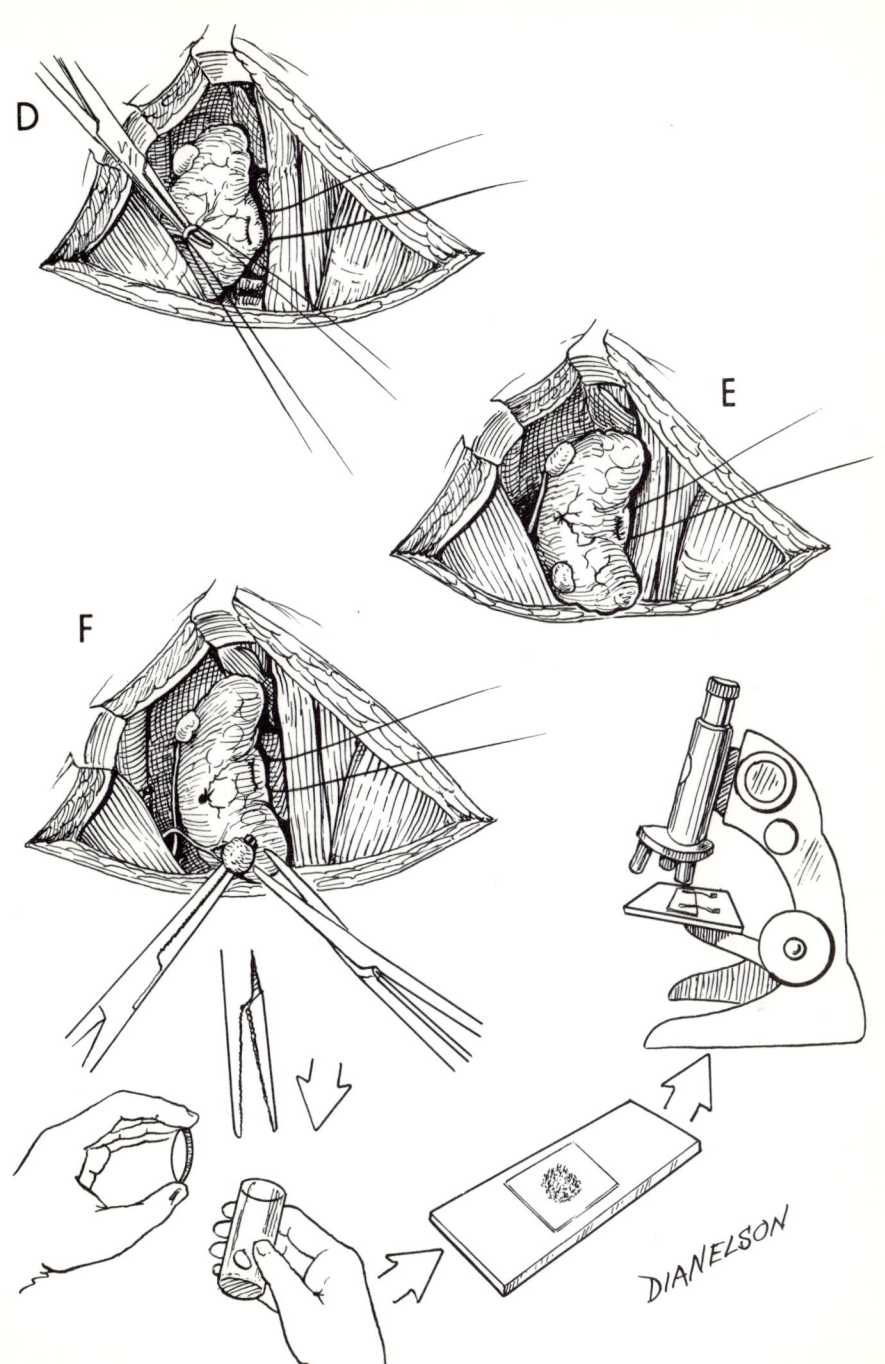

EXTENT OF PARATHYROID TISSUE EXCISION. — The governing principle is to resect all parathyroid tissue except for a remnant that is equivalent to the normal amount of parathyroid parenchyma found in the age group and sex of the patient. The weight of all 4 parathyroids averages 140 mg in adults; it is approximately 130 mg in males and 150 mg in females. Late in childhood fat cells begin to appear in increasing numbers, to the point that approximately one half the cross-sectional area is composed of fat cells by adulthood; in other words, a normal adult has approximately 70 mg of parathyroid parenchyma.

For the reasons stated above the histologic evaluation of all 4 parathyroids for degree of hyperplasia (adenomatous hyperplasia) and fat content is essential before the surgeon decides which glands and how much of each he will resect.

After the surgeon has dissected and estimated the weight of all 4 glands, if possible, and after a frozen-section histologic evaluation has been obtained, the 2 largest glands are resected **(G)**. Then, depending on the size and vascular supply of the remaining 2 glands, he may choose to resect the third gland or one half of each of the 2 remaining glands in such a fashion that approximately 70–100 mg of well-vascularized parathyroid parenchyma is left in situ.

The parathyroid remnant(s) is marked with a metallic clip for future identification. In rare instances, when the vascular supply of 1 of 2 remnants is uncertain, it is preferable not to leave it in situ, but to mince it and to transplant it into the sternocleidomastoid muscle.

CLOSURE. — Before closure of the incision, devascularized portions of the thyroid gland may be excised; although this is not absolutely necessary, it achieves better healing. A drain is usually not required. The strap muscles are approximated with 0000 nonabsorbable sutures **(H)**. Catgut is used to close the platysma **(I)** and the skin is approximated with very fine sutures, alternating with 1/8-in. adhesive paper strips **(J)**. Metallic clips (Michel) are seldom used, for they may leave a chain of pinpoint scars on both sides of the incision, especially if they are not removed by 48 hours after operation.

PLATE 12

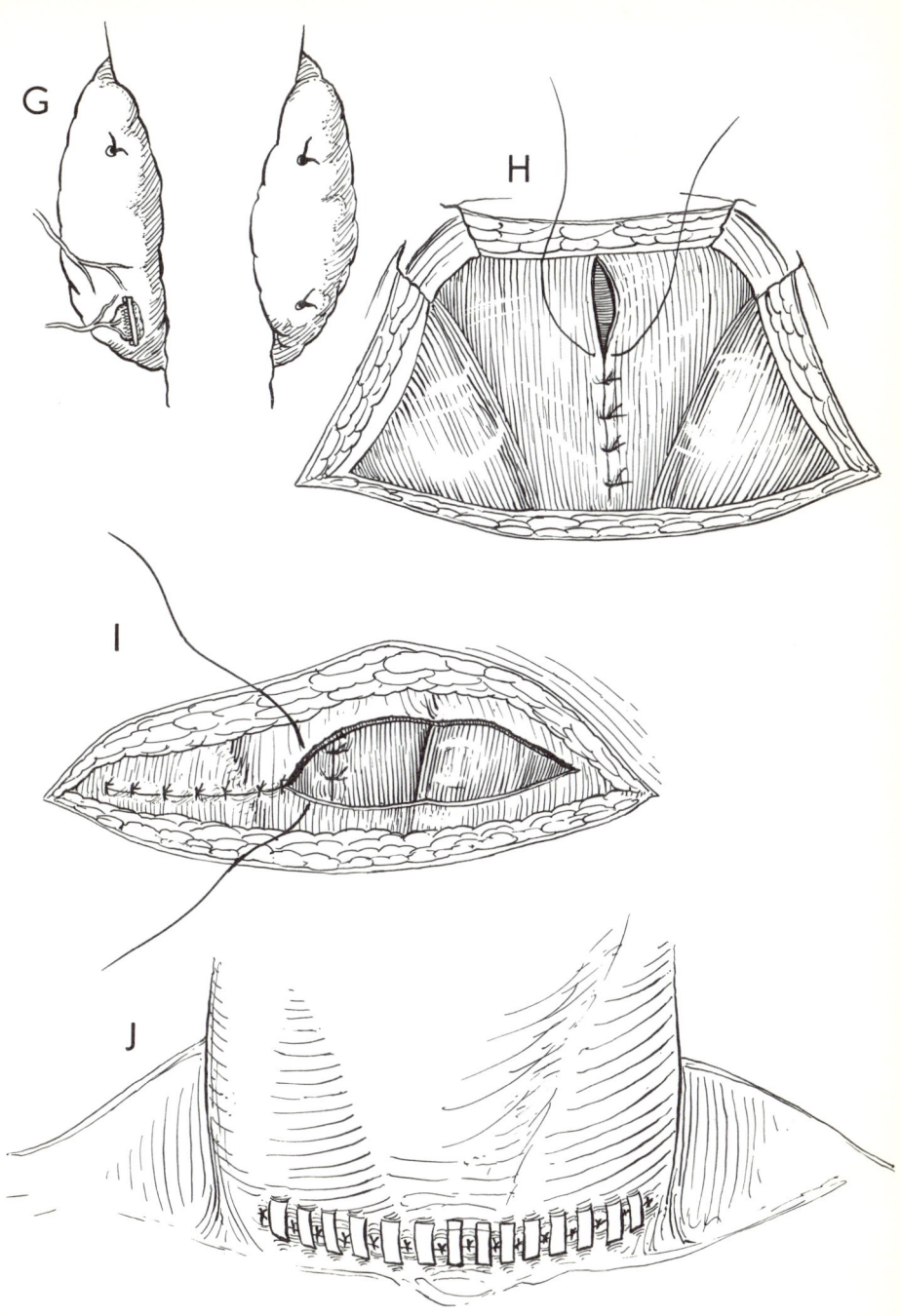

Routine Postoperative Care

The stress of the operation should be minimized as much as possible; opiates, which stimulate spasm of the sphincter of Oddi, must be avoided. Antacids are given preoperatively and postoperatively to buffer acid secretion in the event an ulcer diathesis is not recognized and to neutralize the stimulating effect of gastric acid on pancreatic secretion.

Profound metabolic and clinical changes may be seen following successful parathyroidectomy. Hypocalcemia, if it is going to develop, may not occur for 12–72 hours, presumably because of the prolonged action of PTH and the availability of some PTH secretion from remaining cells. The function of remaining glands or autotransplanted tissue will, however, falter with the onset of edema and associated inflammatory reaction to impaired blood supply. Functional recovery of these tissues may therefore require several weeks or months. Symptoms of hypocalcemia become more noticeable to the patient with the increase in dietary phosphate load once a normal postoperative diet is resumed. During the first week patients may experience bizarre psychologic distress; they and their families should be forewarned that this may develop but reassured that the phenomenon is temporary. The judicious use of sedatives and antianxiety drugs is effective.

The First 24 Hours

Important aspects in postoperative management during the first 24 hours consist of:
1. Airway problems
2. Wound bleeding
3. Acute pancreatitis
4. Accelerated metastatic precipitation of calcium salts in the kidney

Airway problems.—The primary concern for the patient who has undergone any neck operation is the maintenance of an adequate airway. The dual trauma inflicted to the larynx and the vocal cords by parathyroidectomy and by endotracheal intubation leaves little margin for error. A small amount of bleeding that might escape notice if it occurred in the chest or abdomen may trigger a catastrophic chain of events in the neck if it is not detected early and corrected.

For the reasons outlined earlier, precautionary measures must be adhered to. They are presented in chronologic sequence:

1. Neck explorations start at 8 A.M. Thus bleeding, if it occurs, will be manifest by 10 P.M. rather than at 3 A.M.

2. Prior to closure, the wound is irrigated, intrathoracic pressure is increased and all bleeding points (except on the skin) are controlled. It is an unnerving experience to discover a slit in a medium-sized neck vein that had escaped notice and bleeds profusely only when intrathoracic pressure is increased.

3. A very light dressing is used, such as 1 layer of gauze, which allows a full view of the neck and its size by the medical and nursing staff.

4. As soon as the patient is awake in the recovery room, he or she is asked to phonate a high-pitched "e" and to cough. A high-pitched "e" and an effective cough are the best indications of intact and functioning recurrent laryngeal nerves.

5. The patient's head and thorax are elevated to a 30-degree angle during the first 18 hours.

6. From the recovery room the patient is transferred to an intermediate care facility where 1 nurse needs to divide her attention among only 2 or 3 patients. The patients are usually fully awake and ambulatory the evening of operation and will be offered liquid food. The principal reason for placing them in an intermediate care unit is to detect any increase in the size of the neck, airway problems or bleeding at an early stage.

Wound bleeding. — Management of bleeding is handled in the following ways: in an acute emergency, the incision is opened on the ward, the clots allowed to escape and the patient intubated. These steps are seldom necessary. Usually there is sufficient time to transport the patient back to the operating room, where intubation can be done while the surgeon prepares to perform a tracheostomy. The wound is reopened, and bleeding points that can be located are controlled. A soft rubber drain is placed through the sternocleidomastoid muscle into the dissection site and is brought out at the appropriate end of the skin incision. Separate stab wounds are avoided in the neck. Finally, a tracheostomy *must* be done; this precaution is essential, since airway obstruction from laryngeal edema invariably develops within a few hours. There is no known medical means of avoiding laryngeal edema that follows a second intubation and neck re-exploration.

The foregoing complications are seldom if ever seen following simple parathyroidectomies. They may occur following a combination of thyroidectomy and parathyroidectomy.

Acute pancreatitis. — In some series a high incidence of postparathyroidectomy pancreatitis has been encountered. For this reason opiates such as meperidine for the relief of pain are to be avoided, especially since these patients seldom complain of severe pain. Generally they are more distressed by musculoskeletal posterior nuchal and scapular discomfort attributable to positioning on the operating table. This discomfort lasts 1–2 days. Postoperative abdominal pain should be considered an attack of acute pancreatitis until proved otherwise.

Calcium salt deposition in kidney. — Hydration and assurance of a good urinary flow must be maintained pre-, intra- (no catheters, please) and postoperatively, especially during the first 24 hours following removal of hyperplastic parathyroid tissue. Adequate hydration will help to avoid or minimize the precipitation of calcium salts in the renal parenchyma and tubules. Such calcium salt deposition is enhanced by both the decreased flow of urine in the immediate postoperative period (antidiuretic-hormone effect) and by decreased tubular reabsorption of calcium secondary to abrupt relative PTH withdrawal. This latter factor results in transient hypercalciuria, even though serum calcium levels may fall to subnormal values.

The Second 24 Hours

1. Suture removal
2. Check of the vocal cord function
3. Management of hypocalcemia

Skin sutures are removed on the second day and are replaced by adhesive paper strips. The patient may start wearing a cervical collar intermittently for support and comfort.

Hoarseness is most likely due to vocal cord edema from intubation, but can represent a delayed response of injury to 1 or both recurrent laryngeal nerves. Vocal cord paralysis should be observed for at least least 18 months before Teflon injection is considered, since full recovery of function can be expected in well over 50% of patients. For permanent vocal cord paralysis a Teflon injection of the paralyzed cord will help improve voice quality and vocal cord function dramatically.

RESULTS OF PARATHYROIDECTOMY FOR PRIMARY HYPERPARATHYROIDISM

Parathyroidectomy should induce a successful remission of hypercalcemia and most of the symptoms associated with this disease in over 95% of the patients. Fewer than 2% of patients should require mediastinal exploration to locate "true" mediastinal aberrant tumors; fewer than 2% may have parathyroid carcinoma with the possibility of recurrence of symptoms from a local or distant metastasis.

With near-total parathyroidectomy recurrence rates for primary hyperparathyroidism should approach zero. The incidence of permanent hypoparathyroidism and lateral recurrent nerve palsy should be less than 2%.

PATHOLOGY

It is no longer possible to distinguish the classic "adenoma" of yesteryear from hyperplasia. The terms that are gaining acceptance are adenomatous hyperplasia and multiglandular disease. These terms imply that more than 1 parathyroid gland is involved in a given patient. In recent series, where histologic data on 2 or more parathyroid glands are available, the incidence of multiglandular disease has ranged from 25 to 68%. The incidence of a single "adenoma," with atrophy or absence of hyperplasia in the other 3 glands, has dropped to less than 50% in most reports. The incidence of carcinoma is remarkably stable at 2%.

Hypocalcemia of some degree will develop within 72 hours of successful parathyroidectomy. By and large, absence of postparathyroidectomy hypocalcemia means that an insufficient quantity of parathyroid tissue was excised or that the disease was so early in its course and so mild that indications for parathyroidectomy were equivocal, or the diagnosis was in essence incorrect. Hypocalcemia accompanied by normal or low serum phosphorus levels is confirmatory evidence that the catabolic process caused by hyperparathyroidism has been reversed and that accretion of calcium phosphate salts into bone is proceeding at a rapid pace. In patients with severe bone disease (usually associated with a high alkaline phosphatase level) secondary to long-standing or neglected hyperparathyroidism, reversal of the negative calcium balance may be brisk, hence the label of "bone hunger." This form of post-subtotal parathyroidectomy tetany may last for several weeks.

Perioral **(B)** and fingertip **(D)** paresthesias are early symptoms of hypocalcemia. Positive Chvostek **(A)** and Trousseau **(E)** signs are useful bedside tests to detect incipient hypocalcemia. Hypocalcemia can also be anticipated when the response to the urinary Sulkowitch test **(C)** turns negative. Equal quantities of urine and Sulkowitch reagent are mixed. The absence of a precipitate essentially signifies complete tubular reabsorption of calcium, which occurs when the serum calcium approaches 7 mg/100 ml.

Management of Hypocalcemia

Rare episodes of bona fide acute tetany seen in the immediate postoperative period and often precipitated by hyperventilation are best treated with a slow intravenous infusion of 10% calcium gluconate; 2 or 3 10-ml ampules may be required. This solution should be administered into a large vein and given no faster than 2 ml/minute. In patients receiving digitalis, intravenous calcium should be given with great caution and very slowly, preferably with an electrocardiographic monitor, since calcium augments the effect of digitalis and may acutely provoke a digitalis toxic arrythmia.

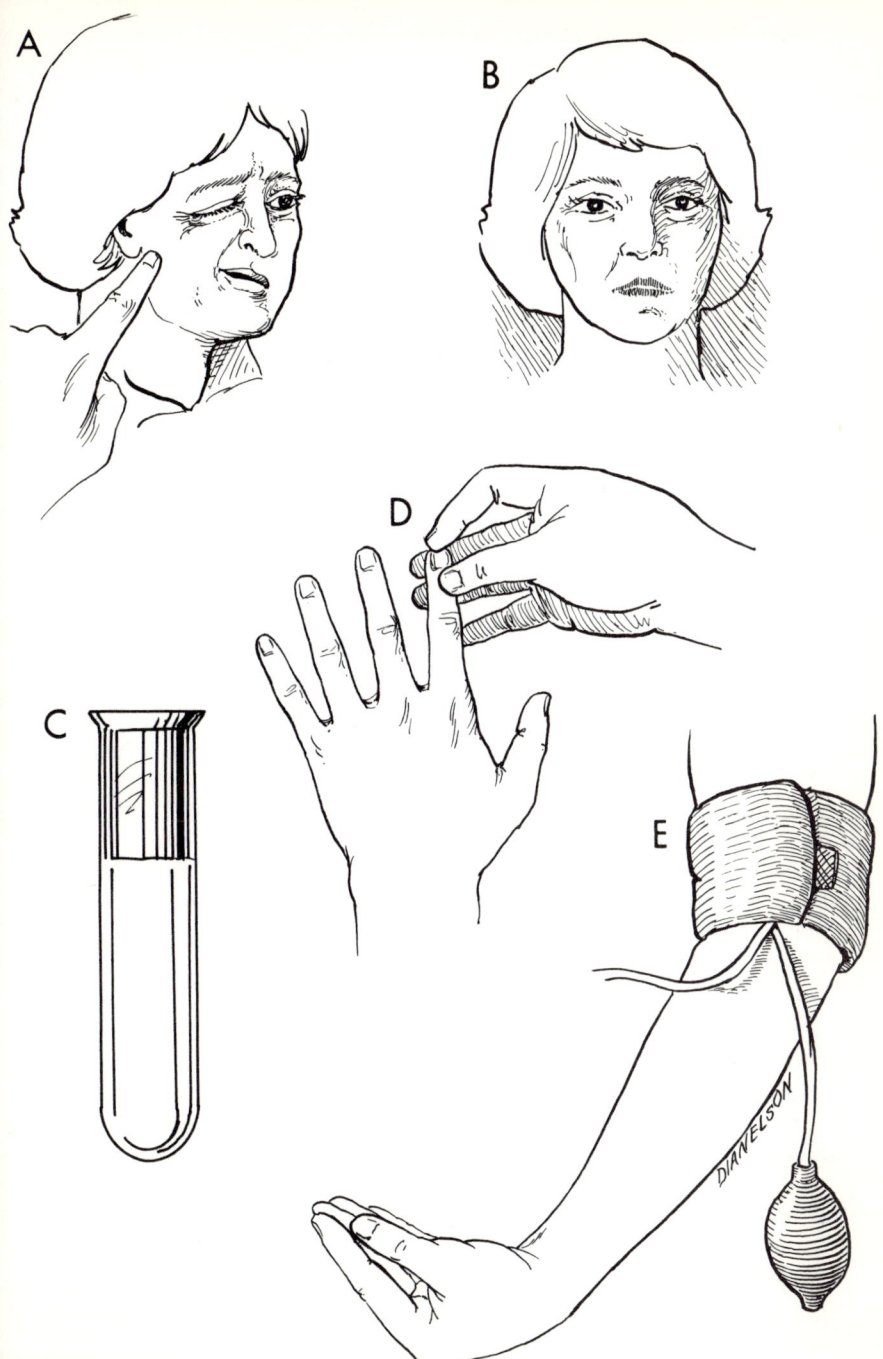

Direct intravenous injection of calcium chloride should seldom be used, as this salt is very irritating to the veins in the concentrations available commercially.

Symptoms of hypocalcemia are generally mild and ephemeral in the majority of patients, who may experience occasional perioral paresthesias, muscle cramps and tingling of the fingertips. These symptoms are aggravated by hyperventilation and/or excessive dietary phosphate intake. Treatment consists of calcium gluconate wafers at a daily dose of 12–16 gm administered orally in divided doses every 6 hours. Exogenous phosphate is restricted by dietary limitation and by the administration of aluminum hydroxide gel, which binds inorganic phosphate in the gastrointestinal tract.

In infrequent instances of prolonged and symptomatic hypocalcemia or repeated episodes of mild tetany, hospitalization is shortened if the patient is started on dihydrotachysterol (AT-10) and calciferol (vitamin D). These two sterols are started simultaneously at respective doses of 0.25 mg every 6 hours and 100,000 units daily. Calcium wafers are added to assure availability of calcium. Dihydrotachysterol gives relief of symptoms within a few hours; there is usually return of serum calcium to the normal range by 24–48 hours. The full effect of calciferol, which mainly enhances calcium absorption from the digestive tract, is not manifest for 10–14 days, at which time the dihydrotachysterol and calcium supplements are discontinued. Thereafter dosage of calciferol can be progressively reduced to 50,000 units daily, a common maintenance dose of vitamin D. As patients differ somewhat in their response to dihydrotachysterol, serum calcium levels should be determined at frequent intervals to detect hypercalcemia. Patients should be alerted to the symptoms of hypercalcemia, such as fatigue, thirst and polyuria, and should contact the attending physician if such symptoms arise between clinic visits.

After a few weeks of normocalcemia on this regimen, the administration of calciferol can be discontinued by reducing the dose over a period of 3 months.

Long-Term Follow-Up in Parathyroidectomy

Once these patients' disease has been corrected and they have fully recovered, it is advisable to evaluate their status at 12-month intervals. In the course of these yearly examinations, they should be screened for recurrence of hypercalcemia and for onset or recurrence of renal stone disease, pancreatitis and hypertension. The accretion of calcium into bone is best evaluated and quantitated by bone density measurements and by conventional x-rays in the rare instances in which osteolytic lesions or severe osteopenia were present prior to operation. These osteolytic lesions (sites of brown tumors) and the lamina dura may undergo dense recalcification.

PARATHYROID AUTOTRANSPLANTATION

In rare instances in which the parathyroid remnant is thought to have an insufficient blood supply, or the patient has had previous surgery and it is known that removal of the entire newly discovered tumor would leave him with insufficient parathyroid tissue, either the remnant or approximately 70 mg of the adenoma is minced and implanted in the sternocleidomastoid muscle or the forearm musculature. These patients are immediately started on 100,000 units of vitamin D daily and 0.25 mg dihydrotachysterol and 4 gm of calcium gluconate wafers every 6 hours. Gradual weaning from sterol support and calcium supplements is achieved over 2-3 months. Autotransplantation of sufficient parathyroid tissue can be expected to yield normally functioning cells in more than 90% of patients so managed.

RE-EXPLORATION AFTER PARATHYROIDECTOMY

A second exploration is indicated in 2 circumstances: (1) when the patient remains hypercalcemic after the first parathyroidectomy, and (2) when hypercalcemia recurs following a variable period of eucalcemia.

Assuming accuracy of the diagnosis of primary hyperparathyroidism, persisting or recurring hypercalcemia means either that insufficient hyperplastic tissue was removed (recurrence rates of 15-100% have been recorded), or that an undiscovered supernumerary gland is present, if 4 glands had been identified histologically at the first operation.

Once the diagnosis of hyperparathyroidism is confirmed again, localization studies are indicated in almost all patients prior to a second operation, especially in cases where all 4 glands were not identified at the first operation.

LOCALIZATION STUDIES.—The simpler localization technics, such as a barium swallow and thyroid scanning, can provide only circumstantial evidence for a parathyroid tumor. The precise localization of an aberrant or overlooked tumor requires a combination of arteriography and venography with sampling of venous blood for PTH immunoassay.

The technics of percutaneous transfemoral and transbrachial catheterization (Plate 14) are used to reach the left and right thyroid arteries, respectively. The dexterity of the radiologists, who are able to catheterize the superior and inferior thyroid arteries and even some of their tributaries (inset), is amazing. Arteriography is at first limited to the side of the missing gland. However, in patients who have had 4 glands identified histologically at the first operation and in whom either the growth of parathyroid remnant(s) or the presence of a supernumerary is responsible for the recurrence, bilateral studies may be required if the study on the first side fails to disclose an enlarged parathyroid. The venous phase of an arteriogram will often delineate the venous drainage of the visualized tumor and simplify the task of venous catheterization and sampling.

[Localization of aberrant or overlooked tumors *continued on page 66.*]

PLATE 14

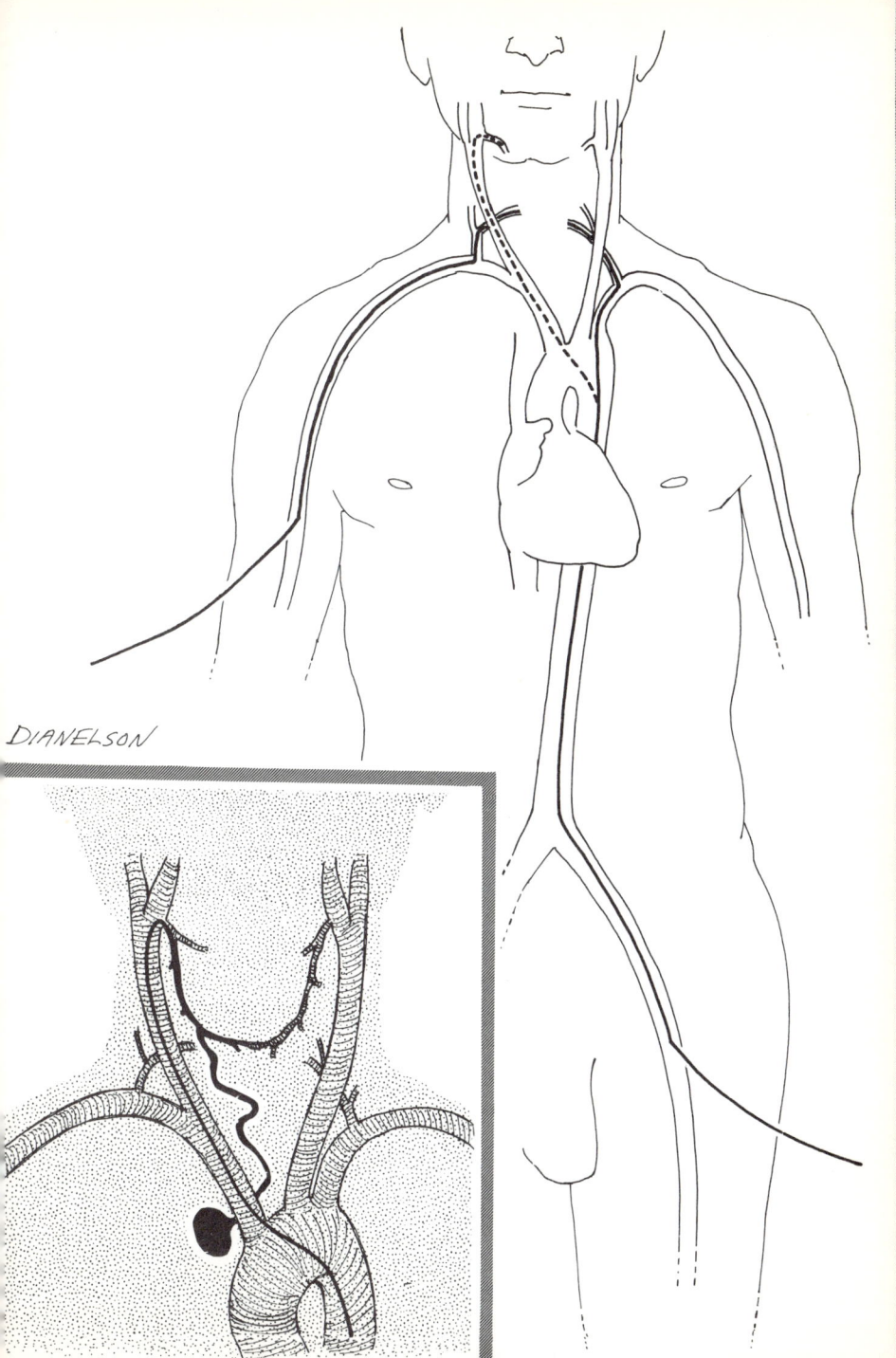

The principal role of transfemoral venous catheterization is to obtain blood samples from the superior, middle, inferior thyroid and innominate veins bilaterally to establish differential PTH levels. The extent and completeness of the study depends upon the skill of the radiologist and the anatomy. In some instances retrograde venography will delineate a tumor (inset). If the radiologist succeeds in catheterizing the vein that drains a visualized tumor and obtains a sample of blood with comparatively high PTH levels, the localization is virtually ironclad.

OPERATIVE TECHNIC.—Re-exploration is a relatively simple task if the tumor has been localized. In the absence of precise localization, both lobes of the thyroid are mobilized and palpated. If PTH data indicate the tumor may be on 1 side, the corresponding thyroid lobe is excised in case the tumor is entirely embedded within the thyroid substance. If this fails, the neck is carefully re-explored (Plate 12), with special attention given to possible ectopic sites within the neck.

If a careful and thorough neck exploration still fails to disclose the aberrant gland, the surgeon proceeds with a median sternotomy. This allows visualization of the superior mediastinum both from the cervical and from the thoracic incisions.

The mediastinal thymic lobes are dissected, excised and examined for intrathymic parathyroid tissue. The retroesophageal space is then dissected and visualized as far down in the chest as is possible. If the missing gland still is not identified, the pleurae must be entered bilaterally to allow visualization of the deeper retroesophageal space and the posterior surface of the trachea behind the carina. This can be more easily accomplished if the azygos vein is divided, and dissection of the posterior mediastinum proceeds from the right side.

If the missing gland is found and is the only known parathyroid tissue remaining in the patient, then a portion of it should be minced and transplanted into skeletal muscle, provided the tissue has gross and microscopic characteristics of a benign tumor.

The danger of injury to the recurrent laryngeal nerves is far greater at the time of the second neck exploration and dissection of the mediastinum than at the first. Normal anatomic tissue planes are obliterated by the first operation, making it imperative that the recurrent laryngeal nerves be identified early and protected during the operation.

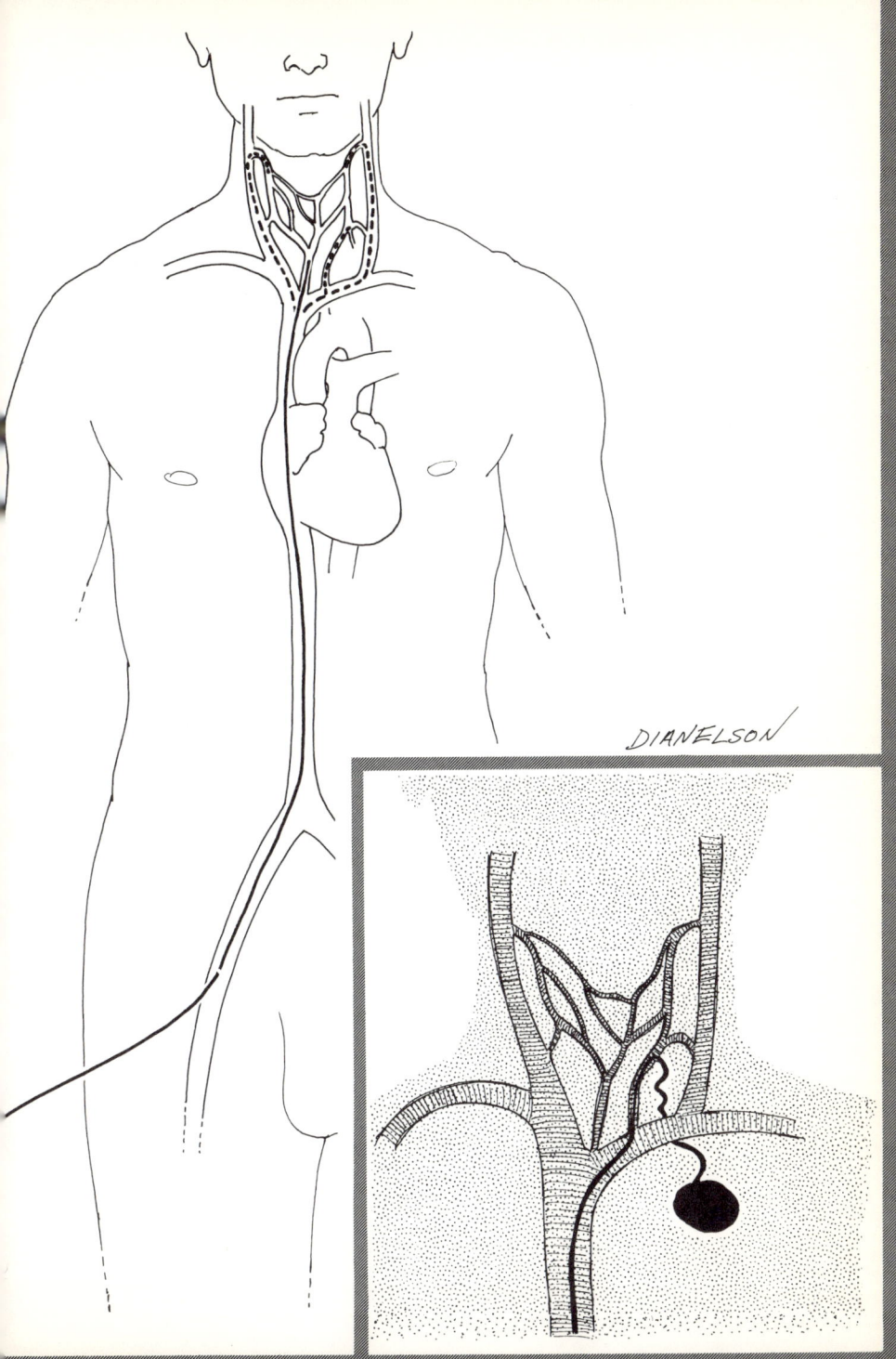

Renal (Secondary) Hyperparathyroidism

Large numbers of patients throughout this country and in many other medical centers outside this hemisphere are being kept alive by means of chronic dialysis. With technical perfections, home dialysis programs and the anticipated marked reductions in dialysis costs, it is safe to predict that the numbers of these patients will increase further. In such patients the hyperphosphatemia and the marked reduction in calcium absorption are very potent stimuli to the parathyroid glands.

It has recently been discovered that the kidney plays a key role in the conversion of vitamin D to 1,25-dihydroxycholecalciferol, the most potent known metabolite with regard to its effect on the absorption of calcium from the gut. In chronic renal insufficiency there is little or no conversion of vitamin D to this metabolite. This may explain the greater susceptibility of anephric patients to renal hyperparathyroidism.

It may well be that within a few years, as more information is gathered, the manipulations of electrolyte concentrations in dialysate, the reduction of serum phosphate with aluminum hydroxide gel and the availability of potent vitamin D metabolites for administration will reduce the incidence of renal hyperparathyroidism.

PATHOLOGY.—It is of interest to note that there is considerable variation in the pathologic findings in renal hyperparathyroidism. Although in most patients all 4 parathyroid glands are uniformly enlarged and may weigh anywhere from 200 mg on up (normal weight 20–40 mg), in some patients only the 2 superior glands or, alternatively, the 2 inferior glands may be enlarged. In others 1 gland may weigh as much as 5 gm while the others weigh less than 200 mg each. The latter example could be explained on the theoretical basis of "tertiary" hyperparathyroidism. The hyperplasia of 2 superior or 2 inferior glands alone is difficult to understand and may provide clues to the pathogenesis of parathyroid hyperplasia.

Chief cell hyperplasia is an almost uniform finding.

DIAGNOSIS AND INDICATIONS FOR PARATHYROIDECTOMY.—
Renal hyperparathyroidism should be suspected in a patient who has been on chronic dialysis for several months and begins to complain of bone or periarticular pain, pruritus and increased lassitude.

"Normocalcemia" in such patients constitutes an abnormal elevation of serum calcium, since in most of these patients the serum calcium level is usually in the vicinity of 7 mg/100 ml. Progressive increase in alkaline phosphatase is a further indication of accelerated bone resorption. Conventional x-rays of the skeleton may disclose a progressive demineralization of the long bones, the spine, the phalanges of the hands and the distal end of the clavicles. The relative prominence of vertebral end-plates contrasted to the resorption of the centrum (rugger-jersey spine) is characteristic of these patients. Periarticular and soft tissue metastatic calcifications are common.

When the serum calcium level rises above 10.5 mg/100 ml, these patients have classic tertiary hyperparathyroidism by definition. This means that even if normal renal function were restored, the hyperparathyroidism would persist, since the parathyroids are regarded as autonomous by this stage.

It has been noted recently that 18–24 months after successful renal transplantation, at least 60% of patients still have hyperparathyroidism. This undermines the previously held belief that once renal function is restored, the parathyroids regress and normal parathyroid function ensues. At this stage of our knowledge, the differentiation between secondary and tertiary hyperparathyroidism is difficult.

The indications for parathyroidectomy in patients on chronic dialysis are few and well defined:

Severe incapacitating bone pain
Severe uncontrollable pruritus
Severe widespread demineralization of the skeleton
Metastatic calcifications
Preparation for transplantation
Hypercalcemia

Parathyroidectomy for Renal Hyperparathyroidism

There are 2 schools of thought in the approach to these patients. Three and one-half (near-total) parathyroidectomy is the operation of choice in most centers; however, some surgeons and nephrologists prefer to do a total parathyroidectomy. There is no question that total parathyroidectomy offers the best chance for cessation and perhaps some reversal of the processes just noted, and permanent remission of symptoms. However, the problem of severe hypocalcemia when a patient's dialysis is delayed, at times when the shunts do not function well and require revision, is a serious drawback. With near-total parathyroidectomy the reversal of the symptomatology may not be as dramatic; furthermore, 10% of the patients may have a recurrence and require a second operation.

A good compromise is near-total (3½) parathyroidectomy with autotransplantation of the remnant into skeletal muscle of the neck or forearm. The transplantation site is marked with metallic clips to facilitate identification for partial or complete excision under local anesthesia in case of recurrence.

The preoperative management is similar to that described for primary hyperparathyroidism, except that these patients must be dialyzed within 16 hours before operation and must be observed closely by the nephrologists.

The technic of the operation is the same except that a soft rubber drain is always left in and brought out through the sternocleidomastoid muscle at the lateral end of the skin incision, no matter how dry the field appears, since large volumes of transudate may flow from the dissected surfaces during the first 24 hours.

The thyroid gland is usually quite firm; the strap muscles adhere to it.

All intake is resumed within a few hours after operation; this includes aluminum hydroxide gel and high doses of calciferol. Phosphate intake is restricted. The day after operation the patient is dialyzed again. Since these patients heal rather slowly, the skin sutures are left in at least 3 days and then replaced with adhesive paper strips, which are left in situ for 2 weeks.

Renal Hyperparathyroidism: Parathyroidectomy [71]

In patients in whom only 2 of the 4 parathyroids are enlarged, those 2 should be removed along with 1 of the other 2 glands. Indeed, if the 2 normal-sized glands have a combined weight that does not exceed 60 mg, the surgeon may choose to leave them both in as remnants, after having established their identity by frozen section.

RESULTS OF OPERATION.—The results are usually dramatic. Bone pain ceases abruptly within the first 48 hours, and patients who have been incapacitated and bedridden are able to ambulate free of pain in short order. Although it is difficult to detect any measurable accretion of calcium in bone, the osteolytic process usually is arrested. Soft-tissue and periarticular metastatic calcifications will resorb in most instances.

In conclusion, parathyroidectomy for renal hyperparathyroidism must be considered a palliative operation. The criteria that govern the indications for parathyroidectomy must be adhered to rigidly.

LONG-TERM FOLLOW-UP.—In renal hyperparathyroidism the best that can be hoped for is the arrest of the progression of bone demineralization and the dissolution of periarticular and subcutaneous metastatic calcifications.

Acute Hypercalcemia with Coma

Rarely, with a sudden rise in serum calcium, a patient may develop intractable vomiting, copious urine output, an atonic bladder, progressive dehydration and life-threatening prostration with severe obtundation. Close surveillance of vital signs, rehydration and the intravenous administration of mithramycin, 25 µg/kg every 24 hours for 3 or 4 days, are measures to be taken immediately. Glucocorticoids are ineffective if the acute hypercalcemia is caused by primary hyperparathyroidism. Intravenous administration of buffered phosphate solutions, although effective in lowering the serum calcium level, carries the serious risk of extensive metastatic calcification by precipitation of calcium phosphate salts within the renal parenchyma. If necessary, hemodialysis should be resorted to. If the diagnosis of hyperparathyroidism is reasonably certain, then one may wish to proceed with parathyroidectomy, which under these circumstances requires little if any anesthesia.

Parathyroid Carcinoma

The diagnosis of carcinoma is suspected by the surgeon at the time of operation when he has great difficulty in mobilizing 1 of the parathyroids, which is bound down firmly by dense collagen bands. This suspicion is further supported by the pathologist when he notes broad fibrous bands crisscrossing the parathyroid parenchyma. However, the number of mitoses and the pleomorphism are not criteria that can be utilized to diagnose malignancy. Actually, most experienced endocrine pathologists will refrain from making a firm diagnosis of carcinoma until nodal or distant metastases have been demonstrated. Perfectly benign parathyroid tumors may show a great deal of pleomorphism, with numerous mitoses.

When a carcinoma is suspected, a more extensive resection, with wide margins of normal tissue, is in order. Frequently it is difficult to identify grossly the malignant tumor as parathyroid tissue. It may have the appearance of a thyroid nodule protruding from the posterior surface of the gland. To ascertain complete excision of the malignancy, near-total parathyroidectomy is imperative in these patients; if hypercalcemia recurs, it will be due in all likelihood to recurrence of the malignancy rather than to continued growth of the other glands, since the other glands, except for the remnant, have been excised. In such an instance of recurrent hypercalcemia a second exploration is justified. If the remnant has not grown or has atrophied, the surgeon is justified, in the absence of detectable distant metastases, in proceeding with an extensive resection of the tissues surrounding the site of the previous carcinoma, even if this means a partial laryngectomy, since recurrent carcinoma of the parathyroids is a lethal disease, even though it can be controlled temporarily with the administration of phosphates and mithramycin. If cervical metastases are encountered, an extensive resection with neck dissection aimed at eradicating the malignancy is in order. The benign parathyroid remnant should be excised to facilitate evaluation of the patient's status with serum calcium determinations in the future. Further recurrence should be treated with phosphates and mithramycin.

The Coexistent Thyroid Tumor

The mass one palpates in the neck of a patient with hyperparathyroidism usually turns out to be a thyroid nodule. There is an apparent increased incidence of thyroid tumors among hyperparathyroid patients. In the course of the parathyroidectomy, the thyroid nodule is removed; if it is benign on frozen section, additional resection is not required.

Thyroid carcinomas other than the medullary variety are treated conventionally by total thyroidectomy and appropriate neck dissection when indicated. Since the extent of resection may compromise the blood supply to any parathyroid remnant, autotransplantation of that remnant will be required in most instances.

Sipple's syndrome (medullary thyroid cancer, hyperparathyroidism and bilateral pheochromocytomas) should be suspected in a patient with hyperparathyroidism and a coexisting thyroid malignancy. This is especially true if there is a family history of the syndrome. When pheochromocytomas are recognized, bilateral adrenalectomy should be performed first. Parathyroidectomy and thyroidectomy are carried out after an appropriate interval for recovery. Following bilateral adrenalectomy, these patients will require superphysiologic doses of cortisone or hydrocortisone during any subsequent operative or other major stress.

Coexistent Hyperthyroidism

The diagnosis of hyperparathyroidism is difficult in the presence of hyperthyroidism, as hypercalcemia and hypercalciuria occur in both diseases. A euthyroid state should be achieved before the diagnosis of hyperparathyroidism is firmly established. The best approach is to treat the hyperthyroidism with radioactive iodine (^{131}I), allow the thyroid gland to atrophy and then proceed with diagnostic evaluation and parathyroidectomy if the diagnosis of hyperparathyroidism is confirmed. Preparation or treatment of the hyperthyroid patient with antithyroid drugs is to be discouraged. These drugs increase the vascularity of the thyroid gland, which is already enlarged and engorged. Although this effect can be reversed with Lugol's iodine and thyroxin administration, a parathyroid exploration would be ill advised in such a setting.

Rebound Hypercalcemia in Recovery Phase of Acute Pancreatitis

Hypocalcemia occurs in as many as 40% of patients with acute pancreatitis. This is probably caused by hypersecretion of hormones, such as glucagon, which have a hypocalcemic effect. There is evidence that this hypocalcemia stimulates the parathyroid glands, with resulting increase in PTH secretion. When this persists during the recovery phase of pancreatitis, it may actually promote transient hypercalcemia. Since the association of hyperparathyroidism and calcific pancreatitis is well known, the first thought that occurs when such rebound hypercalcemia is observed is that the patient is actually hyperparathyroid. In most of these patients, however, this hypercalcemia resolves within a few days and the diagnosis of hyperparathyroidism can be set aside.

When hypercalcemia persists, the patient is allowed to undergo complete recovery from the pancreatitis before any diagnostic procedures for evaluation of possible hyperparathyroidism are instituted. If hyperparathyroidism is ultimately confirmed, parathyroidectomy is indicated. However, prophylactic measures must be taken to reduce the risk of postoperative acute pancreatitis in such patients.

HYPERCALCEMIA AND PANCREATIC MASS

In a patient with hypercalcemia, hypophosphatemia and a pancreatic mass, 2 possibilities must be considered: (1) chronic relapsing pancreatitis (pseudocyst) and associated hyperparathyroidism; (2) a pancreatic carcinoma that elaborates a PTH-like substance. The history and diagnostic procedures to rule out pancreatic malignancy are helpful in differentiating these two conditions. For instance, if the pancreatic mass has been present for a long time, or if there is a long history of alcoholism and relapsing pancreatitis, the chances are that the mass is either a pseudocyst or due to a chronic inflammatory process, which may not have as yet reached the stage of a pseudocyst. A pancreatic mass developing on the heels of an acute pancreatic inflammatory process is most likely a pseudocyst. However, the incidence of pancreatic malignancy in patients with chronic pancreatitis may be higher than in the general population. Furthermore, pancreatic malignancies may trigger attacks of acute pancreatitis by obstructing the ducts.

If after full evaluation, the diagnosis is still uncertain, the abdomen is explored first. In the absence of evidence for a malignancy, parathyroidectomy is done after an appropriate interval. In rare situations the 2 operations may be done consecutively in the same day.

Conversely, if at neck exploration the parathyroids are not particularly enlarged and especially if the hypercalcemia persists after near-total parathyroidectomy, the provisional diagnosis reverts back to pancreatic malignancy and pseudohyperparathyroidism. Deep-seated pancreatic malignancies may be difficult to diagnose even with extensive laparotomy and multiple biopsies. To compound this diagnostic problem, in patients with pseudohyperparathyroidism the parathyroid glands may be hyperplastic.

PSEUDOHYPERPARATHYROIDISM

The list of malignant tumors that elaborate PTH or PTH-like substances and vitamin D-like sterols is a long one. Furthermore, a few benign endocrine tumors secrete PTH-like substances. It has been postulated also that these tumors elaborate substances that stimulate the parathyroid glands, with ensuing parathyroid hyperplasia and PTH hypersecretion.

One of the more difficult problems in the differential diagnosis of hypercalcemia is the possibility of an occult malignancy. In the presence of an obvious malignancy, the diagnosis is pseudohyperparathyroidism until proved otherwise. The primary treatment is directed at the malignancy.

At the current state of the art, immunoassays do not clearly differentiate between PTH emanating from the parathyroids and that emanating from ectopic sources.

When an occult malignancy is suspected but not documented, the history and the degree of skeletal demineralization are important differential determinants. A long history of hypercalcemia and evidence of demineralization of the bones support the diagnosis of hyperparathyroidism. In the absence of these findings and when the common complications of hyperparathyroidism are simply not manifest, a variable period of observation on an outpatient basis and periodic re-evaluations are advisable.

In a patient with breast cancer metastatic to bones and severe hypercalcemia with hypophosphatemia who is on the verge of death from coma, serious consideration should be given to parathyroidectomy. A number of cases have been reported in which the patient whose condition was deemed terminal recovered fully after the resection of large parathyroid glands. The critical determinant in this situation, if the patient has normal renal function, is the presence of hypophosphatemia. The combination of hypercalcemia and hypophosphatemia points to excess PTH, since most breast malignancies do not secrete ectopic PTH; the hypercalcemia they cause is thought to be secondary to the elaboration of vitamin D-like sterols and is usually not accompanied by hypophosphatemia.

HYPERTENSION

There is a surprisingly high incidence of hypertension in primary hyperparathyroidism. This is not related to measurable impairments in renal function. There have been claims that this hypertension may be related to the hypercalcemia. However, correction of the hypercalcemia seems to have little if any discernible effect on the intensity of the hypertension. In some instances, following parathyroidectomy there is a reduction in the antihypertensive medication dose requirements.

Renal Calcareous Disease

Once the hyperparathyroidism is corrected, the progression of renal calcareous disease ceases. Occasionally a few patients will continue to complain of sporadic attacks of renal colic during the first few months following parathyroidectomy. Such episodes are most likely due to residual stones. However, if these attacks persist, either the diagnosis may be incorrect or an insufficient amount of parathyroid tissue may have been resected.

Coexistent Peptic Ulcer Disease

The reported increased incidence of peptic ulcer disease in hyperparathyroidism remains unsubstantiated. However, there is little doubt that hypercalcemia promotes gastrin release and gastric secretion, and that correction of hyperparathyroidism and hypercalcemia leads to the amelioration of duodenal peptic ulcer diathesis. Such patients should be treated with aluminum hydroxide gel antacids in the preoperative and postoperative periods, even if they are asymptomatic.

Pseudogout and Gout

In hyperparathyroidism uric acid levels may be elevated without any symptom of arthritis. After parathyroidectomy these values fall into the normal range.

The relationship between pseudogout and hyperparathyroidism is not clear, except for a reported 30% incidence of hyperparathyroidism in pseudogout. Parathyroidectomy seems to have no influence on the course of pseudogout.

In contrast, patients with gout and hyperparathyroidism seem to be benefited by parathyroidectomy; the acute attacks may be less frequent and long-term treatment, other than dietary measures, may no longer be required.

CHAPTER 2

The Thyroid Gland

A SUPERB EXAMPLE of modern surgical achievement is the development of precise operative indications and refinements in operative technic in the management of thyroid lesions.

In the 1920s and 1930s thousands of thyroidectomies were done for massive goiters produced by iodine deficiency and Graves' disease. The operations for Graves' disease were dramatic. The patient was whisked to the operating theater and had her or his thyroid gland literally whipped out within a few minutes. The complications of thyroid storm, postoperative bleeding and recurrent nerve injury were commonplace in these "horse-and-buggy days." The mortality was appreciable. In the early 1940s, when thiouracil and its derivatives became available, the incidence of postoperative storm was virtually eliminated but bleeding problems were accentuated, since these antithyroid drugs increased the vascularity of the gland to the point that "every capillary became a pumper." It was learned later that this increased vascularity could be reversed effectively by the administration of iodine and/or thyroid hormone.

At approximately the same time antithyroid drugs were beginning to be used extensively, ^{131}I was gaining popularity in the treatment of Graves' disease, especially since antithyroid drugs proved ineffectual in the long-term treatment. The early fears that ^{131}I therapy eventually might produce thyroid malignancies have thus far proved unfounded, at least in the population over age 25. However, high incidences of hypothyroidism have been reported following effective doses of ^{131}I. Hypothyroidism develops insidiously over long periods and is lethal if it escapes diagnosis.

The long-term ineffectiveness of antithyroid drug therapy and the high incidence of hypothyroidism following ^{131}I have forced re-evaluation of thyroidectomy for the treatment of Graves' disease at a time when refinements in anesthetic and surgical technics, combined with preoperative preparation, have reduced the mortality of thyroidectomy for Graves' disease to zero in several large series, with an equally low complication rate. Since the long-term rates of recurrent hyperthyroidism and hypothyroidism following thyroidectomy are less than 5 and 15%, respectively, many internists and surgeons are beginning to prefer thyroidectomy for Graves' disease, especially in the younger age groups.

The treatment of thyroid tumors has also evolved considerably. The extensive, disfiguring and incapacitating operations once done for thyroid cancers are seldom indicated today. The standard neck dissection, an operation originally designed for laryngeal and oropharyngeal malignancies, is seldom done for thyroid cancers. The incidence of recurrent nerve injury and hypoparathyroidism after total thyroidectomy has plummeted.

With modern tools, such as the determinations of circulating thyroxin, triiodothyronine (T_3), thyroid-stimulating hormone (TSH) and microsomal antithyroid antibody titers, refinements in needle biopsies and aspiration cytology and advances in scanning technics, Graves' disease is diagnosed and treated with a greater degree of accuracy, and a high incidence of neoplasia is found in thyroid nodules selected for operation.

Finally, a striking correlation between radiation therapy to the head and neck and subsequent development of thyroid carcinoma has been demonstrated. The "incubation period" for its development varies according to the age at which the x-ray therapy was administered. The shortest incubation periods, of 5–10 years, occur as a rule in patients treated in early infancy for thymic enlargement; the longest, of 25–30 years, have been noted in patients given x-ray treatment for adolescent facial acne vulgaris. In patients who received radiation for tonsillar enlargement at age 3–5, the malignancies develop in their late twenties.

Since the association of radiation therapy and thyroid carcinoma was noted in the mid-1950s appropriate precautions have been taken to protect the thyroid gland, and this etiologic variety of malignancy should cease to exist sometime after the beginning of the next century. We are now at the height of the incidence of malignancies associated with irradiation of the tonsils. That following irradiation for acne should peak in the mid-1980s.

Embryology and Surgical Anatomy

The greater portion, if not all, of the thyroid tissue that will form the follicular elements arises as a median diverticulum of the endoderm of the floor of the primitive pharynx. This diverticulum soon forms a small bilobed structure attached to the buccal cavity by a narrow stalk, the thyroglossal duct, which eventually becomes obliterated. With further development this duct elongates and the bilobed structure becomes more pronounced, descends into the neck and joins on each side ventral components of the fourth pharyngeal pouch. There is no doubt that these ventral elements are intimately related to the development of the thyroid gland; they are sometimes referred to as the "lateral lobes" and are thought to be the source of the parafollicular C cells that secrete calcitonin. However, there is histochemical evidence that these C cells may well be derived from the neural crest and are part of the neuroendocrine system.

In regard to "lateral aberrant" thyroid elements, the authors are convinced that they exist and derive from the fourth pouch.

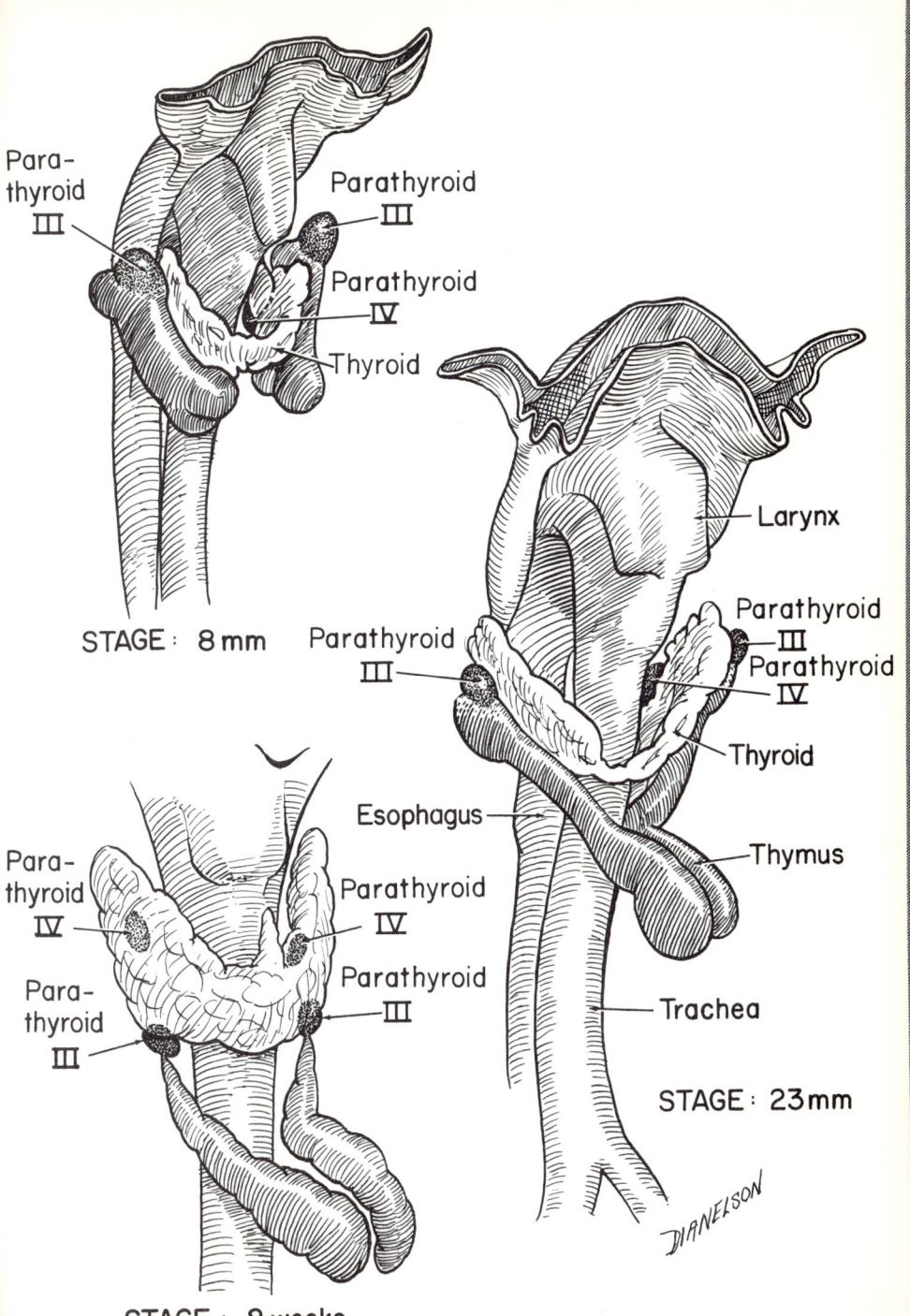

Thyroid Gland: Ectopic Tissue

Aberrant thyroid tissue has been described along the course of the thyroglossal duct, in the superior anterior mediastinum, where it may derive its blood supply from intrathoracic vessels, and within the upper esophagus and trachea. In the cervical region isolated nodules of normal thyroid tissue are quite common, lateral, superior and inferior to the main body of the thyroid gland. These may be chronically inflamed and contain germinal centers of lymphoid tissue and striated muscle.

Truly intrathoracic, usually superior-anterior mediastinal ectopic thyroid tissue and tumors, with a blood supply arising from intrathoracic vessels, are rare occurrences.

A problem arises when a few follicles of normal thyroid tissue are found within the capsule of cervical lymph nodes in the presence of a histologically benign thyroid nodule. The consensus is that those follicles do not respresent metastases, provided the follicular cells appear normal and the follicles are limited to the periphery of the lymph node in a circular or wedge-shaped pattern. Such ectopic tissue is found not only in the presence of thyroid nodules, but also when the gland is entirely normal to painstaking histologic examination.

Finally a word should be said about struma ovarii, a rare occurrence of thyroid tissue in an ovarian teratoma. The term is best reserved for teratomas in which thyroid tissue is the main component. Although rare instances of thyrotoxicosis and malignancy with peritoneal metastases have been reported, thyroid tissue in struma ovarii seldom functions.

PLATE 17

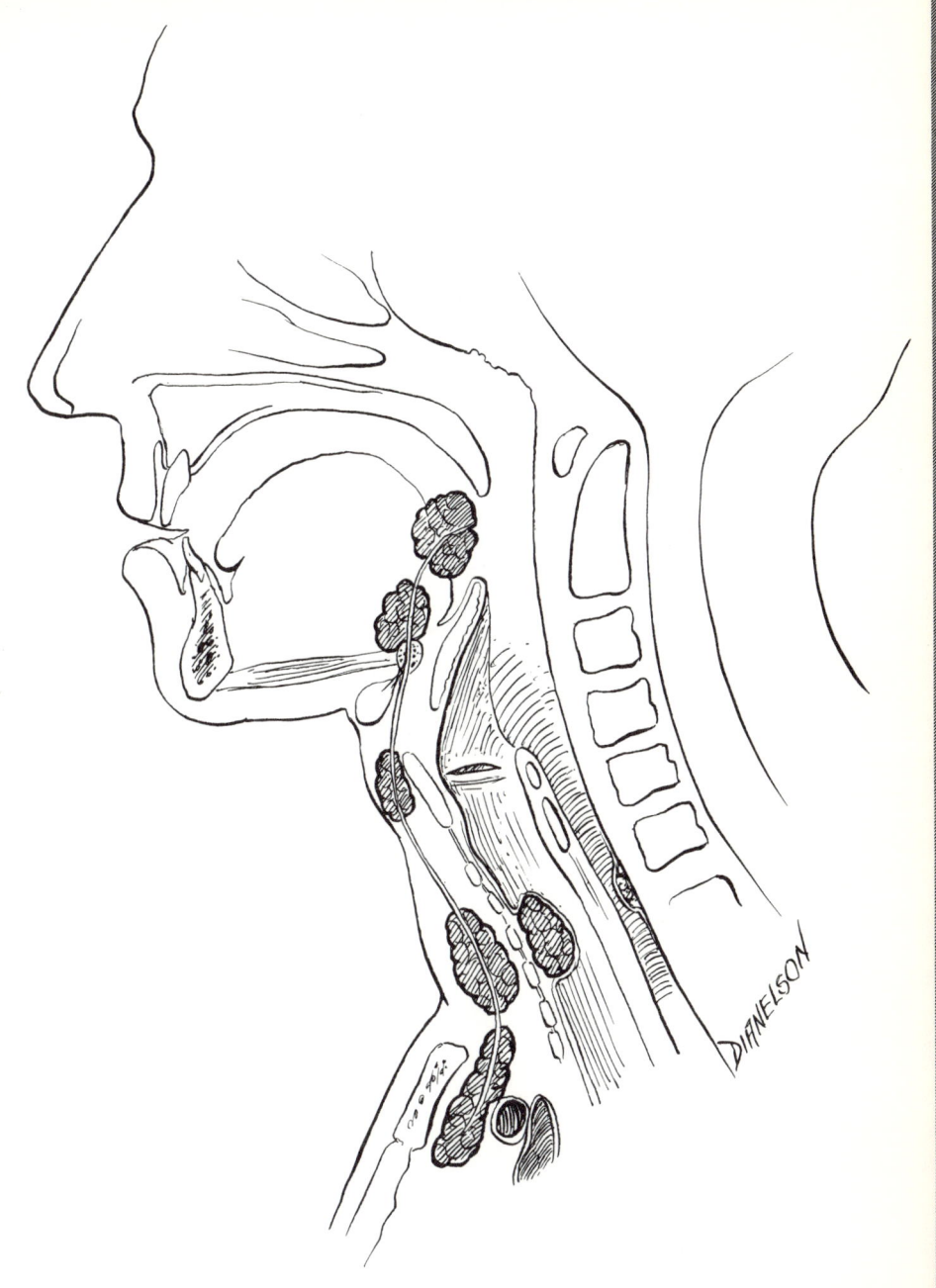

Thyroid Gland: Surgical Anatomy

In operations on the thyroid gland, there is no margin for error. Detailed knowledge of the anatomy, especially the relationship of this gland to the parathyroid glands and laryngeal nerves, is of crucial importance.

The superior and inferior thyroid arteries are derived from the external carotid arteries and the thyrocervical trunks, respectively. The superior and middle thyroid veins drain into the jugular, whereas the inferior veins and the thyroidea ima drain into the innominate veins.

The external branch of the superior laryngeal nerve is closely related to the superior thyroid vessels, especially to their medial branches, which supply the cricothyroid muscles. The recurrent laryngeal nerve bears a relationship to the inferior thyroid artery. It courses obliquely on the right and longitudinally on the left.

The inferior parathyroid glands (III) have variable locations and may be embedded in the thymus. The location of the superior glands (IV) is less variable; they are usually located near the point where the recurrent laryngeal nerves burrow under the lower border of the inferior pharyngeal constrictor muscle and penetrate the cricothyroid membrane (see Plates 4 and 5).

Plate 18 depicts the muscle and cartilage relationships, the arterial supply and the important nerves of this area. Venous drainage is not shown.

PLATE 18

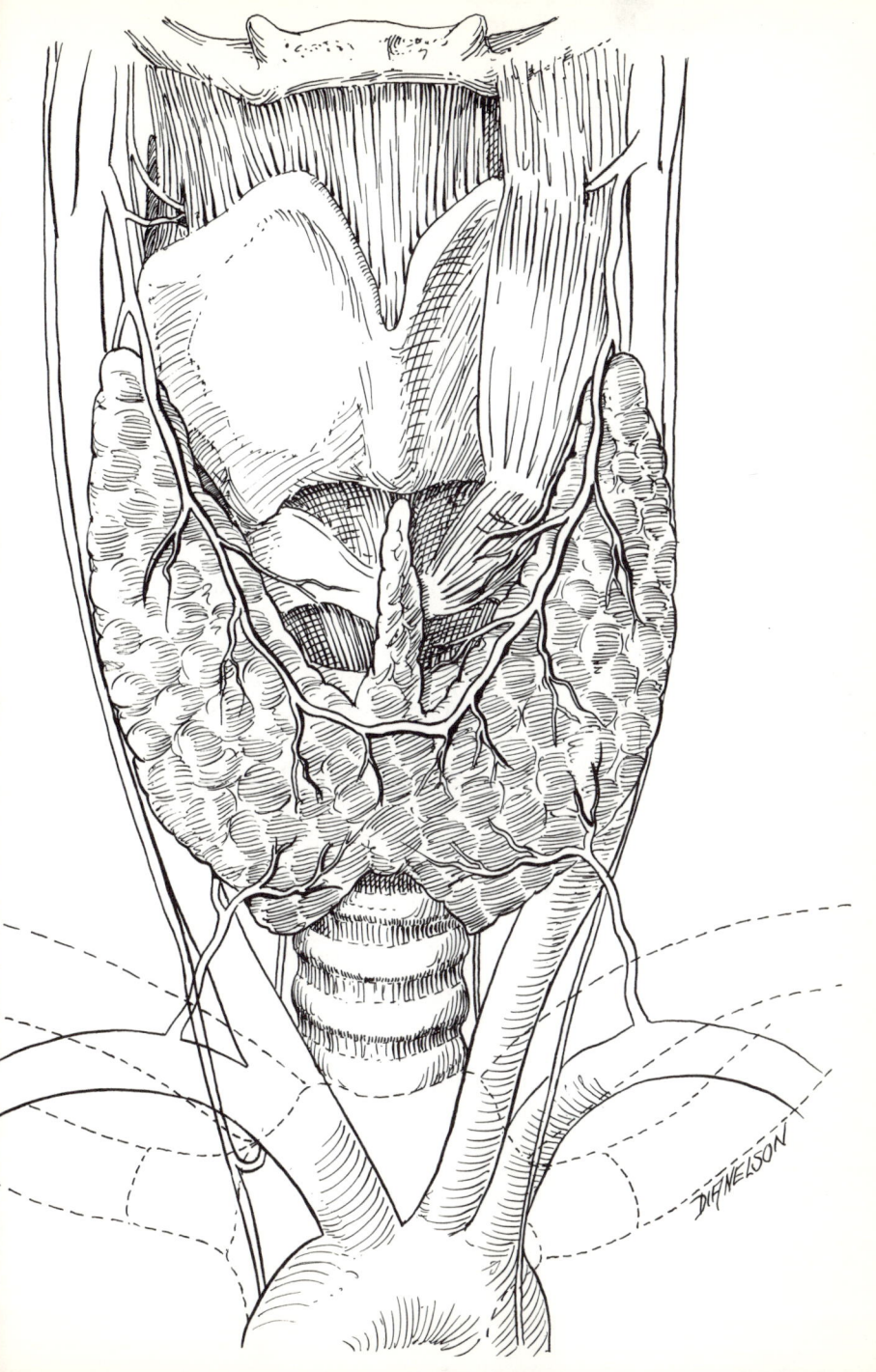

Pathophysiology from the Surgical Viewpoint

The thyroid gland remains the bread and butter of the endocrine surgeon; the results he obtains in thyroid operations are the measure of his technical skill and knowledge, which should include a keen understanding of thyroid physiology, pathology and pathophysiology.

The surgeon is mainly concerned with the therapy of patients with Graves' disease, toxic adenomas, nontoxic adenomas and carcinomas.

THYROTOXICOSIS

GRAVES' DISEASE.—The etiology of Graves' disease is unknown. It is regarded as an autoimmune disease. Circulating TSH levels in these patients are usually low or undetectable; however, they may have elevated titers of a 7S gamma globulin produced as an antibody to thyroid tissue and termed long-acting thyroid stimulator (LATS). The thyroid gland is diffusely enlarged and very vascular, to the point that many patients have a bruit over their glands. The administration of thyroid blockers such as propylthiouracil produces further increases in size and vascularity of these glands, secondary to the stimulation of rising TSH titers. Varying degrees of exophthalmos and pretibial myxedema are manifestations of Graves' disease that are not found in other forms of thyrotoxicosis.

TOXIC MULTINODULAR GOITER (PLUMMER'S DISEASE).—This is a disorder in which hyperthyroidism develops in a background of long-standing multinodular goiter. The elevations of serum thyroxin are usually mild. The diffuse and uneven uptake of ^{131}I is not altered by TSH or exogenous thyroid hormone administration. These findings suggest that the hyperfunctioning areas are autonomous. Whether this autonomy is endogenous in the thyroid or depends on LATS is not known. However, pretibial myxedema and exophthalmos, which are thought to be related to LATS, are not a feature of this disease. Cardiovascular manifestations such as tachycardia and atrial fibrillation tend to predominate. It has been suggested that many of these patients have T_3 toxicity, which may be the reason for the mild elevations of thyroxin (T_4) and the predominance of cardiovascular manifestations and emotional lability. This disease is best treated with ^{131}I.

Toxic Adenoma

A third form of hyperthyroidism is produced by 1 or more autonomous adenomas arising in an otherwise intrinsically normal gland. Usually the adenoma is single and suppresses the uptake of ^{131}I by the remainder of the gland; LATS is not present in the circulation of these patients, and TSH is suppressed. However, exogenous TSH will "light up" the rest of the gland when it is administered prior to a second ^{131}I scan. Toxic adenomas occur in a younger age group than do toxic multinodular goiters; for this reason, and also because the remainder of the gland is not vascular and may even be atrophic and because a number of these nodules have proved to be malignant, the treatment of choice is operative.

Thyroid Tumors

As a rule, benign and malignant tumors of the thyroid do not secrete appreciable quantities of thyroid hormones and have a low uptake of iodine in comparison to normal thyroid tissue. For this reason, they will be relatively "cold" on scans. However, a few malignant "hot" nodules have been described; a number of these have produced toxic symptoms and have suppressed the uptake of ^{131}I by the normal portions of the gland.

Cold nodules that are colloid cysts can be differentiated from benign and malignant tumors by the use of ^{75}Se-selenomethionine scanning. Both benign and malignant tumors have a high turnover of amino acids such as methionine and therefore are warm on selenomethionine scanning, whereas colloid cysts are still cold.

While any appreciable quantity of normal thyroid tissue (2 gm or more) remains in the patient, it is unlikely that ^{131}I scanning will disclose metastases, since the normal thyroid tissue will have a much greater affinity for ^{131}I. Occasionally the ominous finding of patchy and faint ^{131}I uptake in the gland, with uptake in cervical lymph nodes, will be observed. This indicates that most of the normal thyroid tissue has been destroyed by either tumor invasion or coexisting chronic thyroiditis.

Medullary carcinomas of the thyroid, which constitute approximately 5% of thyroid malignancies, are of particular interest to the endocrinologist, since they secrete large quantities of calcitonin and may be associated with other endocrine tumors, such as parathyroid tumors and pheochromocytomas. In spite of the hypersecretion of calcitonin, only 1 case of concomitant hypocalcemia has been described. In general, the high levels of circulating calcitonin produced by these tumors elicit a compensatory hyperplasia of the parathyroids with hypersecretion of PTH and resulting normocalcemia. In the early stages of medullary carcinomas, when the thyroid may be normal to palpation and scanning and circulating calcitonin levels are normal, the administration of intravenous calcium or pentagastrin may provoke an abnormally pronounced rise in circulating calcitonin. This test is particularly useful in screening the family members of patients with proved medullary cancer, since these tumors have a high familial incidence.

Nontoxic Diffuse and Multinodular Goiters

Diffuse hyperplastic goiters are thought to result from an inadequate synthesis of thyroid hormones secondary to a variety of causes such as congenital defects in the biosynthesis of thyroid hormones and nutritional factors, which include dietary deficiencies of iodine or the intake of goitrogens. It is the current belief that these diffusely hyperplastic glands under the fluctuating stimulus of thyrotropic hormone undergo cycles of involution and nodular hyperplasia and eventuate in the all too common multinodular nontoxic "colloid" goiters.

Thyroid Tumors

Thyroid tumors are divided into 2 categories: benign and malignant. One of the most taxing responsibilities of the surgical pathologist is to differentiate between benign and malignant thyroid tumors on frozen section. In some instances, even with permanent sections, the diagnosis is difficult to reach. In Hürthle cell tumors a histologic differentiation between malignancy and benignity cannot be made until metastases are demonstrated.

Thyroid Tumors: Classification

The importance of a correct diagnosis at the time of operation is more than academic, since thyroid malignancies have a high propensity for multicentricity and therefore require a total thyroidectomy as the "minimum" operation.

The main difficulty revolves around pure follicular tumors, since to most pathologists the presence of papillary structures is pathognomonic of a malignancy. Medullary, clear cell and anaplastic cancers are diagnosed with relative ease. The accompanying classification is designed to aid the surgeon in making decisions relative to operative indications and extent of resection during the course of thyroidectomy.

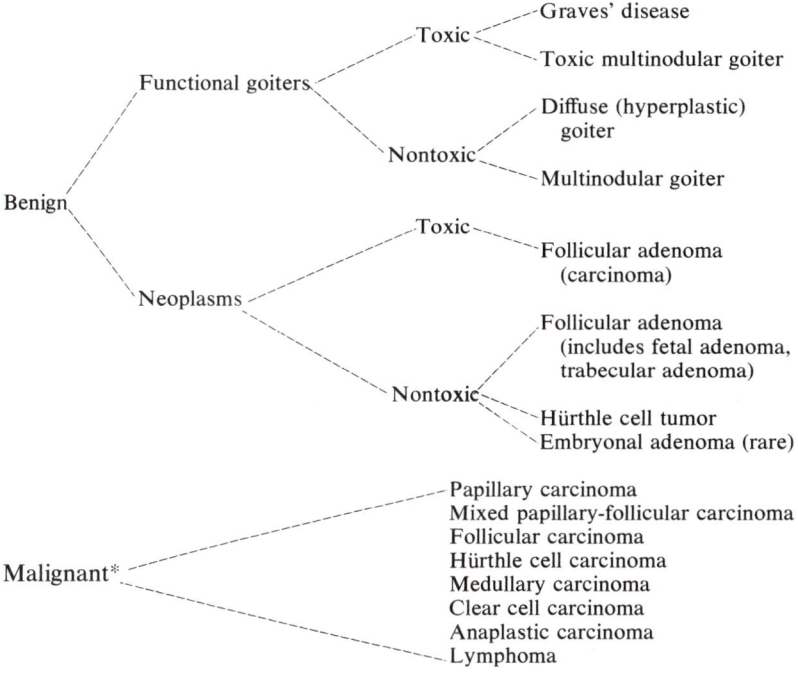

- Benign
  - Functional goiters
    - Toxic
      - Graves' disease
      - Toxic multinodular goiter
    - Nontoxic
      - Diffuse (hyperplastic) goiter
      - Multinodular goiter
  - Neoplasms
    - Toxic
      - Follicular adenoma (carcinoma)
    - Nontoxic
      - Follicular adenoma (includes fetal adenoma, trabecular adenoma)
      - Hürthle cell tumor
      - Embryonal adenoma (rare)
- Malignant*
  - Papillary carcinoma
  - Mixed papillary-follicular carcinoma
  - Follicular carcinoma
  - Hürthle cell carcinoma
  - Medullary carcinoma
  - Clear cell carcinoma
  - Anaplastic carcinoma
  - Lymphoma

---

*These malignant tumors are listed in the order of increasing degree of malignancy, except for the lymphoma.

CLINICAL EVALUATION

In the evaluation of thyroid tumors, the first order of business is to determine the thyroid status of the patient and to institute the appropriate therapeutic measures in case of hypo- or hyperthyroidism prior to full evaluation. Fortunately, the great majority of patients with thyroid tumors are euthyroid.

The indications for the excision of toxic adenomas and massive tumors, especially in the presence of tracheal compression, are clear.

In the selection of patients with cold nodules for operative intervention, a number of factors that increase the possibilities of neoplasm are considered. It is generally accepted that, if the chances of malignancy are 20% or greater, thyroidectomy is indicated, barring medical contraindications. The following factors increase the possibility of malignancy:

1. With a documented history of radiation exposure in infancy, childhood, adolescence and young adulthood in a patient with a thyroid nodule, the incidence of malignancy is 40-70%.

2. Sex. Thyroid tumors have a predilection for female patients. However, the presence of a clinically solitary nodule per se in a male constitutes an indication for operation.

3. Age. Although follicular and papillary carcinomas are distributed evenly throughout all age groups in adults, anaplastic and medullary carcinomas have a peak incidence in the sixth, seventh and eighth decades.

4. A history of rapid growth.

5. A familial history of thyroid malignancy, or of neoplasia in the same patient.

6. Physical characteristics. A clinically solitary nodule, a fixed, hard tumor, suspiciously enlarged and firm cervical nodes, paralysis of a vocal cord and evidence of distant metastases to the lungs or bones are all suggestive findings.

7. Scans. Although a number of malignant, "hot" nodules have been reported, most adenomas and carcinomas of the thyroid are cold on ^{131}I scans. On ^{75}Se-selenomethionine scans a number of adenomas and carcinomas are warm or hot, in contrast to colloid nodules, which remain cold.

8. Hashimoto's thyroiditis. The incidence of carcinoma in these patients has been reported to be as high as 25%.

9. Suppression of TSH. A misconception that still prevails is that if a nodule undergoes involution after suppressive doses of desiccated thyroid or thyroxin, it does not require excision. This concept is misleading and dangerous, since tumors most apt to show regression with TSH suppression are the papillary and mixed cancers. It has been shown that during the course of long-term suppressive therapy in patients with nodules thought to be benign, metastases have appeared.

10. Pre-existing tumor. Another misconception is that a tumor known to have been present for several years is most likely benign. This is not the case. The length of time nodules subsequently proved malignant have been known to be present ranges from a few months to 40 years, with an average of 6 years. This is not surprising, since these are inherently slow-growing malignancies.

As a general rule, thyroidectomy is advised to all patients with clinically solitary cold nodules. This yields a 30–40% incidence of malignancy. The significance of the clinically solitary nodule is puzzling, since at operation or in the surgical pathology laboratory other nodules are usually found in the case of benign tumors, and multiple foci of malignancy in instances of carcinoma.

Histologic Diagnosis Short of Operation

NEEDLE BIOPSY OF NODULES.—The pathologic diagnosis of a thyroid nodule is frequently difficult, even under the best circumstances when the pathologist is in possession of the entire tumor and the surrounding lobe. It is nearly impossible to differentiate a malignant from a benign follicular tumor when working with a sliver of often architecturally distorted tissue. The main applications for needle biopsies are:

1. To confirm the clinical diagnosis of Hashimoto's thyroiditis in a patient with an enlarged nodular thyroid in which a particular nodule may be more prominent.
2. To diagnose papillary and anaplastic carcinomas.

ASPIRATION CYTOLOGY.—With the use of very fine needles to obtain cells from thyroid nodules and/or adjacent lymph nodes, claims of a high degree of accuracy in the selection of patients for thyroidectomy have been made. Papillary, anaplastic and medullary carcinomas can be detected relatively simply by this technic. However, the differentiation between follicular adenomas and carcinomas may be difficult and unreliable; this is not important, since benign neoplasms should be excised as well in view of their propensity to degenerate into malignancies, especially the anaplastic variety.

Thyroglossal Duct Anomalies

The most common anomaly of the thyroglossal duct is a cyst. On rare occasions, cultures of these cysts may give positive results for a variety of organisms, including the tubercle bacillus.

Lingual thyroids are rare. It is important to determine by scanning whether any other thyroid tissue is present before their excision.

Only a few carcinomas in lingual thyroids and thyroglossal duct cysts have been reported in the world literature. The reported malignancies associated with lingual thyroids have been of the follicular and anaplastic varieties, with the expected results from such tumors. On the other hand, almost all reported carcinomas found in the infralingual thyroglossal duct anomalies are of the papillary variety, with its usually good prognosis.

Indications for Thyroidectomy

BENIGN DISEASE.—*Graves' disease.*—Some years ago, with the advent of ^{131}I, the therapeutic approach to Graves' disease began to swing away from resection. The widespread use of ^{131}I in all age groups, including young children, resulted in a number of complications, the most prevalent being a high and rising incidence of myxedema. A number of reports of thyroid malignancies in patients who received ^{131}I in childhood have appeared. With the improvements in preoperative, operative and postoperative management of these patients and with the excellent results of resection, the pendulum is swinging back toward operative management in the younger age groups.

Toxic adenoma.—Since a number of malignancies have been reported in toxic adenomas, resection after a euthyroid state has been achieved is the preferred choice. Large doses of ^{131}I will also effect a cure without damaging the remainder of the thyroid gland, since it is suppressed and will take up very little ^{131}I.

Other benign conditions.—Deviation, compression and constriction of the trachea, obstruction of the thoracic inlet, tracheomalacia, compression of the recurrent nerve(s), compression of the innominate veins and difficulty in swallowing are all indications for operative intervention in otherwise benign conditions such as chronic thyroiditis, toxic or nontoxic multinodular goiters and diffuse goiter. Anomalies of the thyroglossal duct tract such as protruding or enlarging lingual thyroids and thyroglossal duct cysts should be excised.

MALIGNANT DISEASE.—Exploration is advised when the clinical evaluation indicates that a given patient falls into a group with an appreciable incidence of thyroid malignancy; the term "appreciable" will have different meaning in different centers. As an example, the incidence of malignancy in the patients we operate for what we consider clinically solitary nodules fluctuates between 25 and 40% in any given year.

The factors that seem to increase the incidence of malignancy in thyroid tumors have been listed under Clinical Evaluation. In addition, the siblings of patients with medullary cancers may have normal circulating calcitonin and no physical abnormalities of the thyroid, while harboring medullary cancers. Provocative tests produced by the administration of intravenous calcium or pentagastrin may elicit an abnormal rise in calcitonin and lead to the detection of unsuspected medullary cancers.

Preoperative Management

The preoperative management of patients with thyrotoxicosis, especially patients with Graves' disease, mainly consists of achieving a euthyroid state with blocking agents and an involution of the gland to a firm consistency with the concomitant administration of TSH-suppressing doses of thyroxin. The entire process may take several months.

It is desirable to place the patient with thyroid nodules or tumor on TSH suppression for 2 months before operation. This usually causes a shrinkage of the normal portions of the thyroid and frequently of the tumors, and therefore facilitates dissection of the thyroid gland, the recurrent nerves and the parathyroids. In addition, the malignant cells released into the circulation during dissection are less likely to "take" when TSH secretion is suppressed.

Patients should stop smoking 1 month before operation. In case of upper respiratory infection the operation is postponed.

Patients with inflamed, tender thyroglossal duct cysts are treated with antibiotics. Operation is not done until several weeks after the inflammation has subsided.

The anesthesia, positioning and incision are the same for all the operations on the thyroid gland itself. A very light plane of anesthesia, with endotracheal intubation, is preferable. In a professional singer a pharyngeal airway is substituted for endotracheal intubation.

The patient's neck should be positioned with precautions to avoid excessive hyperextension **(A)**. The head and torso are elevated at an angle of 30 degrees. The legs are also elevated to avoid pooling of blood in the lower extremities. An effective way of draping the head is to pass an orthopedic stockinet over the hair and forehead, to place 2 sterile towels under the head and to fold the upper towel over the chin of the patient, thus covering the endotracheal tube. This towel can be fixed to the chin with an adhesive spray; this avoids the use of towel clips or sutures on the face or chin.

PLATE 19

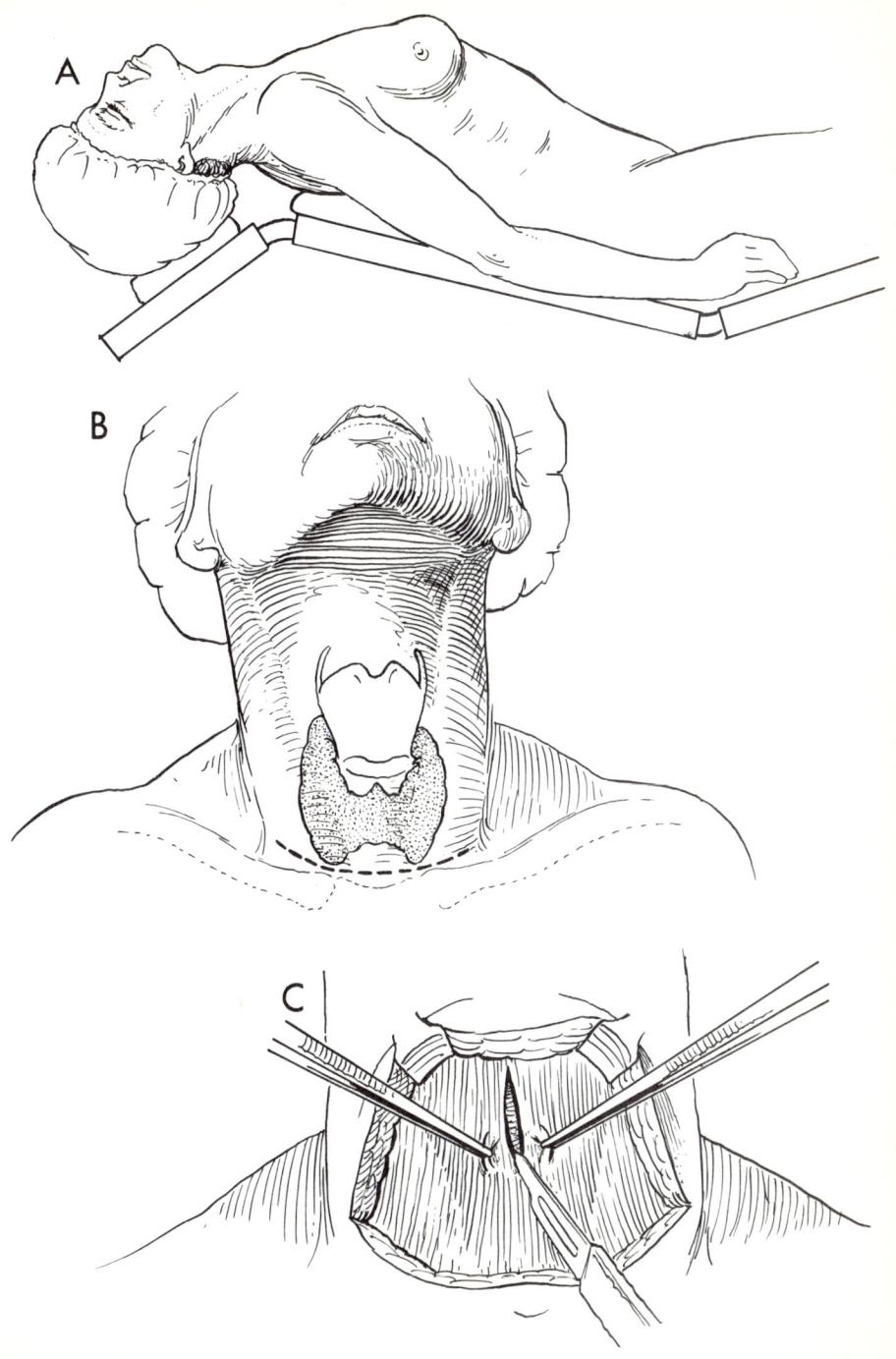

Excision of Thyroid Nodule

The incision is outlined with a string, and measured in both directions from the midline to assure symmetry (**B**). A needle impregnated with methylene blue is used to mark various points on either side of the incision line; this facilitates accurate closure of the incision, which is made in such a fashion that the scar will fall just above the clavicles when the patient is sitting up in a natural position.

The skin incision is carried down to the platysma. It is important *not* to cauterize or impart undue trauma to the edges of the skin incision, since this contributes to excessive scarring and hypertrophy of the scar. For the same reasons the incision should be long enough to avoid excessive stretching during the dissection. The platysma is incised. The skin flaps are developed by separating the platysma from the strap and sternocleidomastoid muscles. The dissection is carried to the notch of the thyroid cartilage rostrally and to the clavicles caudally.

The strap muscles are divided in the midline (**C**) and retracted laterally; on occasions it will be necessary partially to divide the sternothyroid muscles transversely to expose the superior thyroid vessels; branches of the superior thyroid vessels to the sternothyroid muscles are dissected and divided between ligatures in this process.

There are only 2 principal indications for the excision of nodules. First, when a nodule is of such proportions that it compresses the trachea, its excision is considered an adequate operation provided there is no suspicion of malignancy.

The other indication for the excision of a nodule is the situation in which a lobectomy has been performed on one side for a nodule that is benign on frozen section, and another nodule is discovered on the contralateral side. If the second nodule is also benign, the operation is terminated. If the second nodule is malignant, the remaining portion of the lobe is excised and the adjacent lymph nodes are examined.

The excision itself is a rather simple procedure. The approach is shown in **A** and **B**. Once the strap muscles are dissected and both lobes of the thyroid partially exposed, the middle thyroid veins are divided between ligatures. This will permit gentle dissection and

[Closure *on page 98.*]

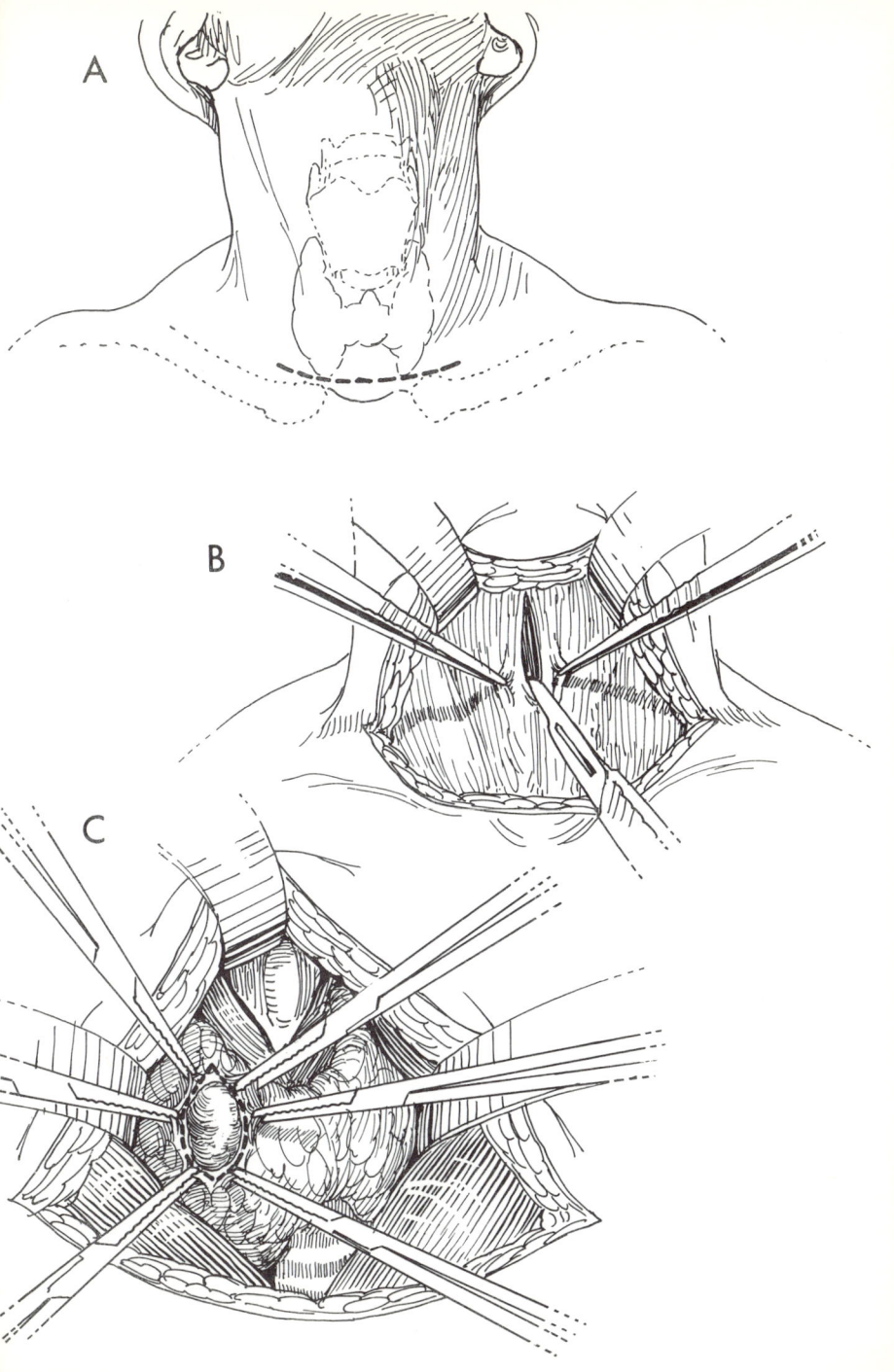

PLATE 20

Excision of Thyroid Nodule

inspection of the posterior aspects of the gland, with forward rotation. At this point gentle dissection is carried along the carotid sheath and in the superior mediastinum in search of enlarged lymph nodes for frozen section examination, to establish a diagnosis of malignancy if possible.

Hemostats are placed on grossly normal thyroid parenchyma to outline the extent of the resection (C). The nodule is enucleated with sharp dissection if it is surrounded by a thick capsule and if there is an identifiable cleavage plane. If this is not possible, the nodule is excised with sharp dissection with a surrounding rim of normal thyroid tissue.

Hemostasis is achieved with suture-ligatures (D). Precautions are taken to place the stitches *within* thyroid parenchyma and thus avoid inadvertent injury to the recurrent nerve.

The incision is closed with great care to achieve a cosmetic result. Furthermore, the strap muscles and the platysma must be well approximated to avoid a continuous scar that would bind the trachea to the skin. This would impair swallowing, as traction would be placed on the skin of the neck by the upward movement of the trachea with each act of deglutition.

The strap muscles are approximated with fine nonabsorbable sutures. The platysma is closed with interrupted fine catgut (E); the knots are inverted. The skin is closed with 6-0 interrupted nylon, at 8 mm intervals. The first sutures are placed on the blue dots for proper alignment. One-eighth inch adhesive strips are placed between the skin sutures (F). These sutures are removed in 48 hours, the adhesive strips in 10 days. Two weeks after the operation the patient is instructed to massage the scar with cold cream at least twice a day for several weeks to prevent its binding to the strap muscles and trachea.

DRAINS.—Soft rubber drains are indicated only when there is a large dead space, when hemostasis is less than absolute or when a large surface of the thyroid has been transected, as in bilateral subtotal resection for Graves' disease. The drain is placed on the surface of the remaining thyroid tissue or in the dead space and passed through an opening fashioned in the sternocleidomastoid muscle between the sternal and clavicular heads. It exits at the lateral end of the skin incision. The drain is usually removed within 24 hours; a suture, placed in the operating room, is now tied to achieve good approximation of the skin edges.

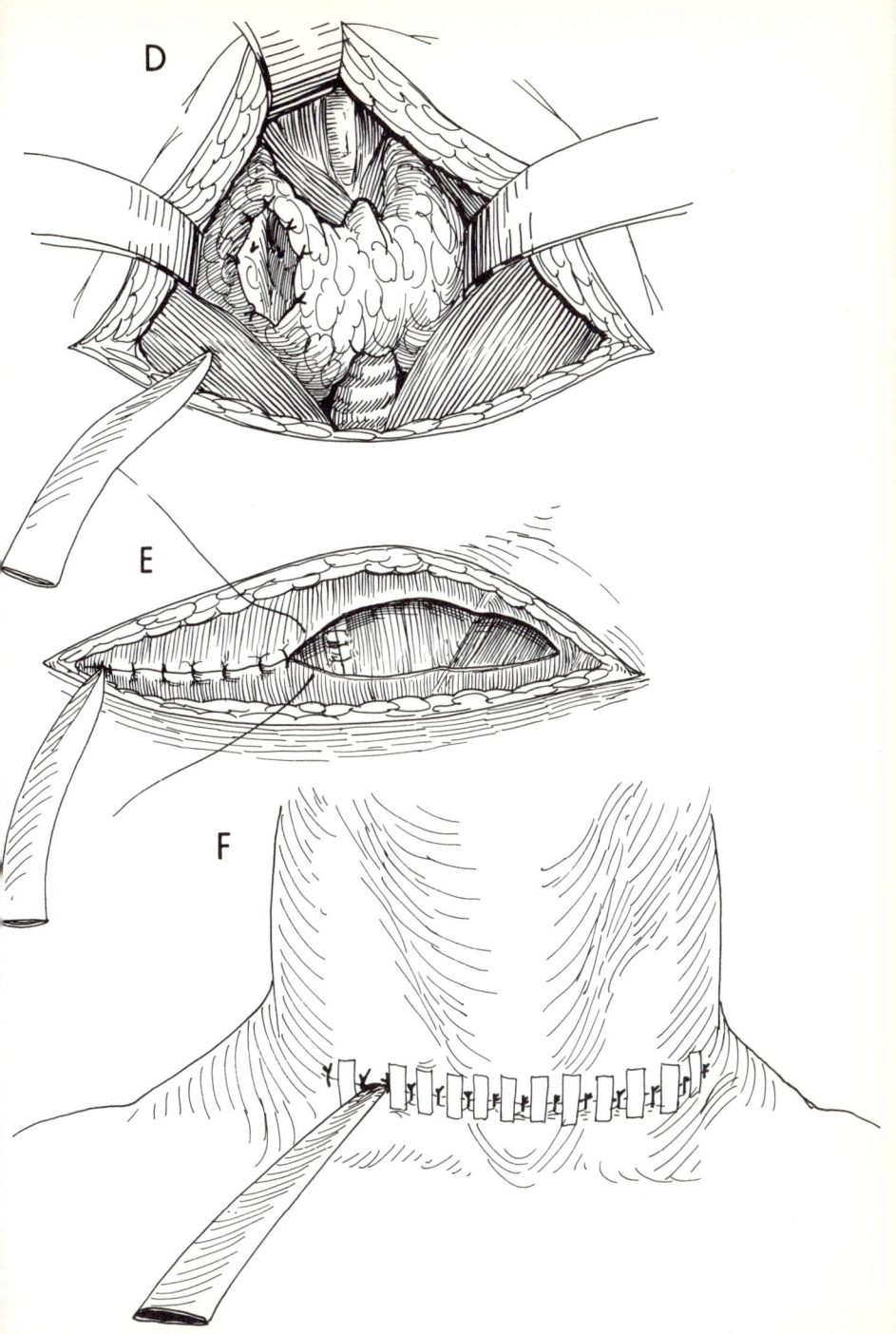

Thyroid Lobectomy

This is the operation of choice for patients who have clinically solitary nodules.

Once the thyroid is exposed **(A)**, the middle thyroid vein and superior vessels are divided between ligatures **(B)**. A suture-ligature is placed in a normal portion of the body of the thyroid **(C)**; this facilitates medial traction and exposure of the posterior surface. The cricothyroid space medial to the superior vessels is developed. Branches to the cricothyroid muscle, coursing transversely perpendicular to the main superior trunks, may have to be divided before the cricothyroid space is developed. To avoid injury to the external branch of the superior laryngeal nerve, these vessels are ligated and divided individually. Once the superior pole is dissected, the lobe is reflected medially and cephalad **(D)**.

Before dividing the inferior vessels, the recurrent laryngeal nerve should be located **(C)** and partially *(very gently)* dissected for 2 reasons: (1) to avoid injury to this nerve, which usually bears a relationship to the inferior thyroid artery, and (2) to locate the superior parathyroid (IV), which usually lies on the cephalic end of this nerve where it penetrates the cricothyroid membrane. The left recurrent nerve runs longitudinally in the tracheosophageal groove, whereas the right courses obliquely. Once the inferior parathyroid is located, the remainder of the excision of the lobe is a simple matter except for a short vein that runs directly medial to the recurrent nerve **(D** and **E)**. This can cause a great deal of troublesome bleeding it it is not dissected and ligated. Frequently this vein is accompanied by a hornlike projection of the thyroid between the recurrent nerve and the cricoid cartilage. Some manipulation and gentle lateral traction of the recurrent nerve may be necessary to excise that projection of the thyroid gland. When some residual thyroid tissue is noted in postoperative scans, inadequate excision of that portion of the gland is very likely the cause. Sharp dissection is usually necessary to separate the remainder of the thyroid from the underlying cartilaginous structures **(E)**. The isthmus and the pyramidal lobe are usually included in a lobectomy. The parathyroids are preserved in situ or are autotransplanted if their blood supply is deemed inadequate (Plate 22).

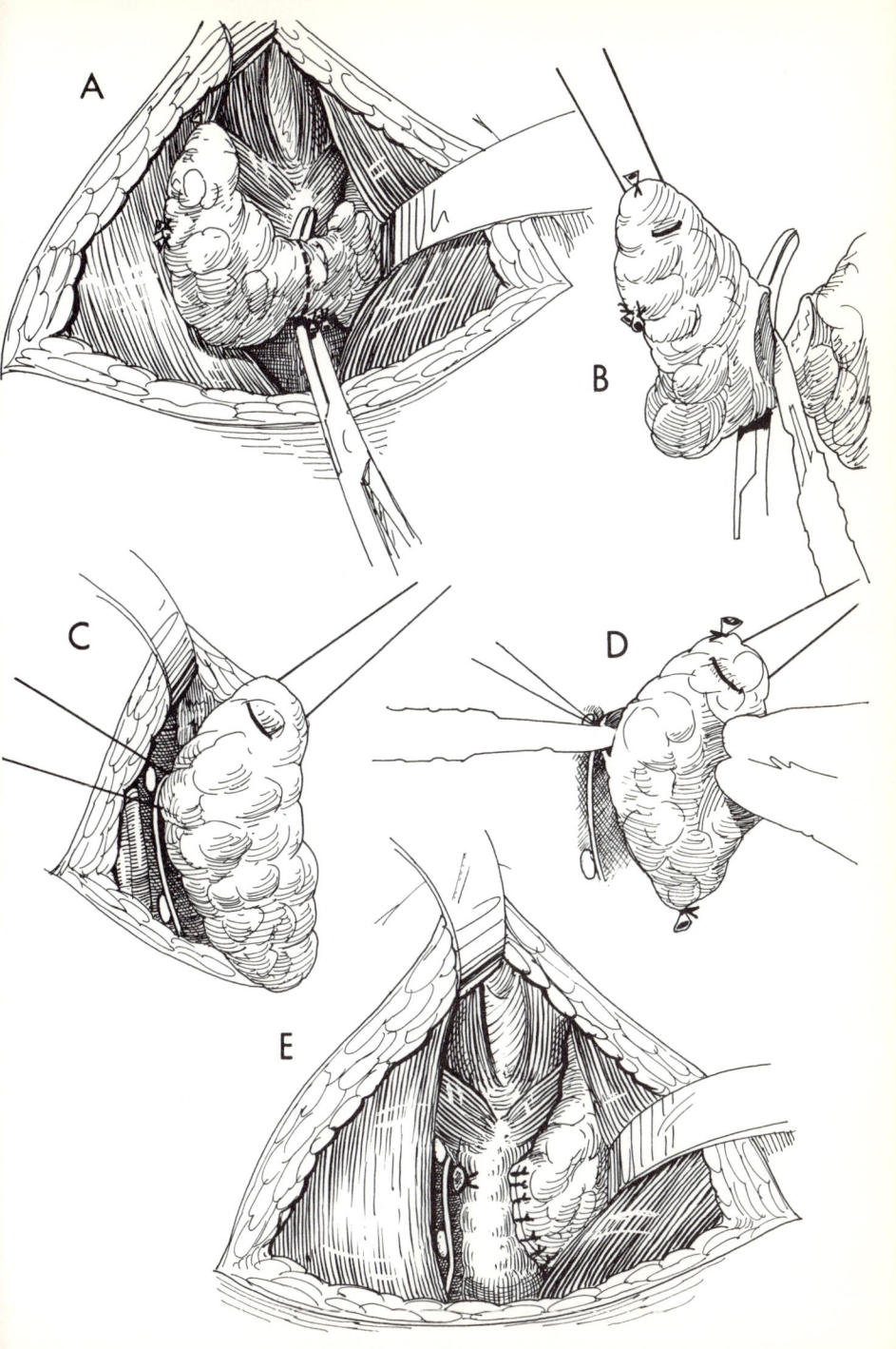

In patients with a history of radiation therapy to the head and neck and in other instances where total thyroidectomy is indicated, the operative procedure described for lobectomy (Plate 21) is done bilaterally. Both recurrent nerves are identified.

With the complete or near-complete excision of the entire thyroid gland **(A)**, both recurrent nerves are exposed after having been partially dissected, especially in their most cephalad segment in the region where they plunge through the cricothyroid membrane; frequently it may be impossible to resect the last remaining segment of thyroid tissue medial to the recurrent nerve at this point.

In total thyroidectomy the preservation of the parathyroid glands is of paramount importance since this operation may lead to the impairment of the vascular supply of the parathyroids. Each of these glands should be identified grossly and the identity confirmed by frozen section of a small fragment. If they are at some distance from the thyroid, within the thymus or the superior mediastinum, they should be preserved in situ. More frequently they are adherent to the thyroid and lose their blood supply during thyroidectomy. To preserve parathyroid function, they are minced into fine pieces and autotransplanted into a pocket fashioned in the ipsilateral sternocleidomastoid muscle **(B)**. The transplantation sites are marked with metallic clips **(C)**.

PLATE 22

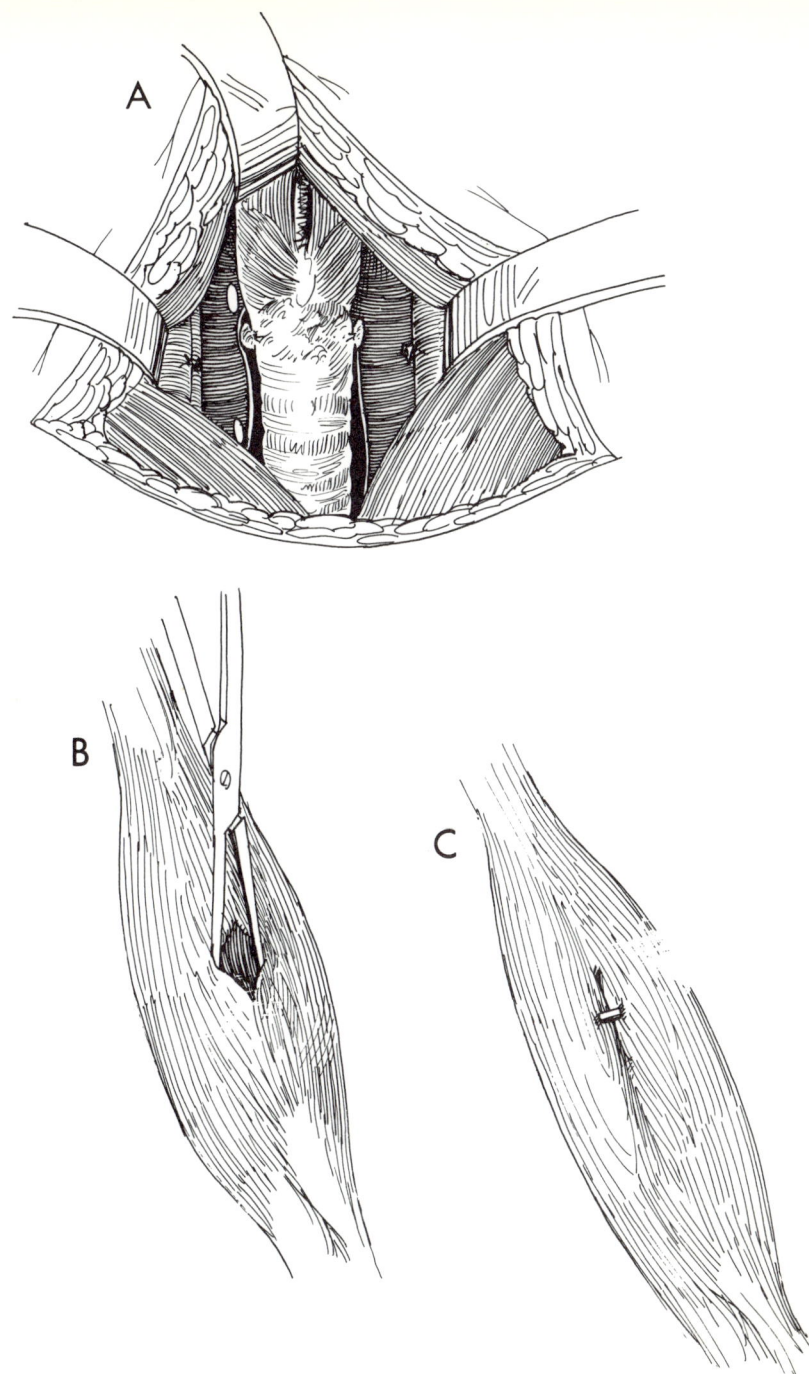

Chapter   *Page*

    Total Gastrectomy in Management 190
    Diarrheogenic Islet Cell Tumors (Pancreatic Cholera,
        WDHA Syndrome) 204
    Glucagonoma(s) 205
4. The Adrenal Gland 206
    Steroidogenesis and Control of Secretion 207
    Embryology 208
    Anatomy and Histology 210
    Cushing's Syndrome 212
    Aldosteronism 218
    Masculinizing, Feminizing and Nonfunctioning Tumors 222
    Pheochromocytoma and Other Amine-Producing Tumors . . . 223
        Causes 223
        Adrenal and Extra-adrenal Locations 224
        Neuroblastomas and Ganglioneuromas 226
        Medullary Cancer of the Thyroid 227
        Clinical Features of Pheochromocytoma 227
        Synthesis and Degradation of Catecholamines 228
        Diagnosis of Pheochromocytoma 230
        Treatment of Pheochromocytoma 230
    Operative Approaches to the Adrenal Glands 234
        Anatomic Considerations 234
        Abdominal Transperitoneal Approach to Right Adrenal . . . 236
        Abdominal Transperitoneal Approach to Left Adrenal . . . 238
        Thoracoabdominal Incision 246
        Posterior Thoracolumbar Approach 248
        Flank Approach 258
5. The Future of Endocrine Surgery 260
    Index 263

In the course of a total thyroidectomy, when the diagnosis of carcinoma has been made histologically, a thorough exploration of the nodal basins **(A)** is done and enlarged nodes excised to determine the presence of metastases. The ipsilateral nodes closest to the tumor are usually involved first. If the tumor is in the isthmus or pyramidal lobe, metastases may be found in the midline pretracheal Delphian or sentinel nodes.

In the presence of nodal metastases, a modified neck dissection on the ipsilateral side along with the excision of accessible nodes on the contralateral side and in the superior anterior mediastinum is indicated. The accessible portions of the thymus are also excised. Extension of the low anterior cervical incision into the supraclavicular space **(B),** on both sides if necessary, will provide more than adequate exposure **(C).**

The purpose of a neck dissection for thyroid cancer is to excise the groups of lymph nodes that drain the thyroid. Although in most instances nodal metastases are confined to one side and the midline, metastases to contralateral nodes occur with sufficient frequency to warrant a limited lymph node excision on the side contralateral to the neck dissection.

Conversely, neck dissection for thyroid cancer is not an en bloc cancer operation such as the procedures designed for laryngeal malignancies. The biologic nature of the slow-growing thyroid malignancies does not warrant an en bloc dissection, which would entail the resection of the larynx, the esophagus and the carotid arteries. Furthermore, cosmetic and functional considerations have popularized the modified neck dissection, in which the sternocleidomastoid muscle is detached from the clavicle and sternum to facilitate the neck dissection, but is preserved and reimplanted at the completion of the operation. The function of this muscle is thus preserved and the contour of the neck is maintained.

[Total thyroidectomy with neck dissection *continued on page 106.*]

PLATE 23

LYMPHATICS

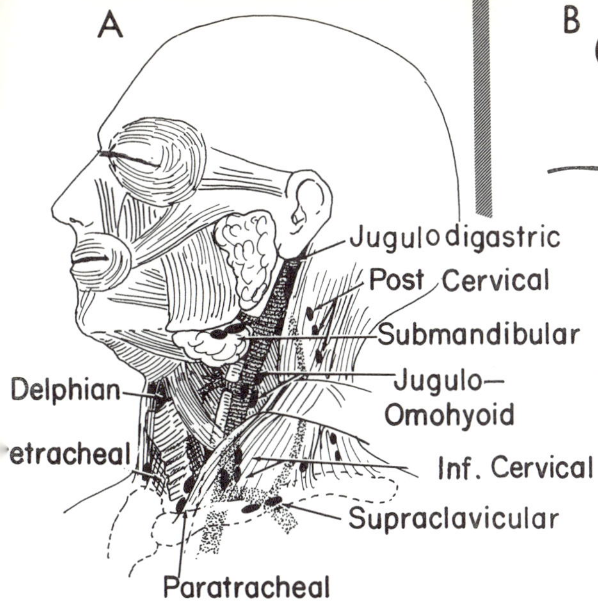

A

- Jugulodigastric
- Post Cervical
- Submandibular
- Jugulo-Omohyoid
- Inf. Cervical
- Supraclavicular
- Paratracheal
- Delphian
- etracheal

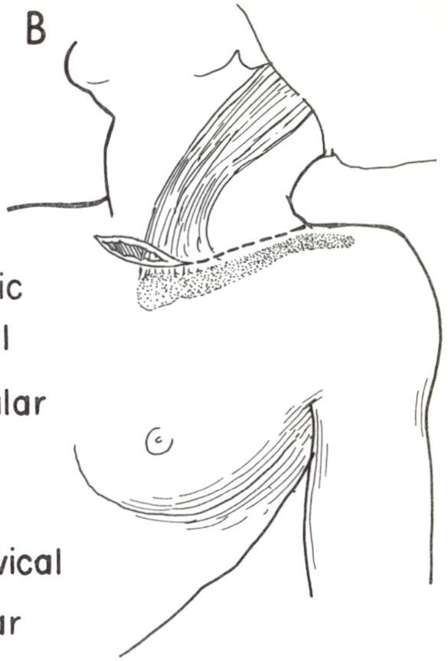

B

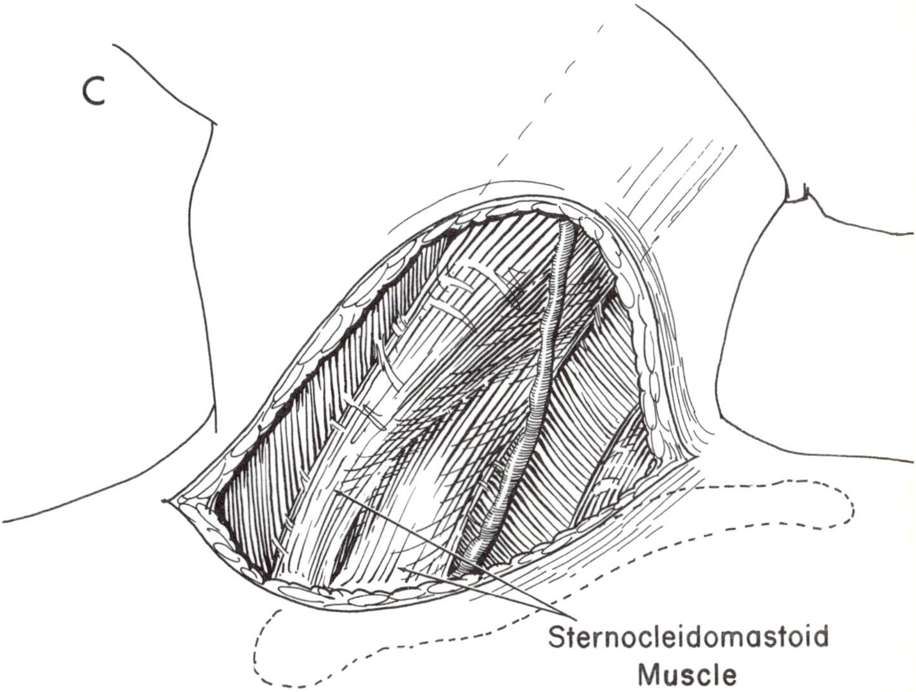

C

Sternocleidomastoid Muscle

Total Thyroidectomy with Neck Dissection

When the decision to proceed with a neck dissection has been made, the incision is extended laterally into the supraclavicular region, almost to the acromioclavicular joint. The flaps are developed further. In a patient with a long, thin neck a countertransverse incision in the submandibular fold may be necessary to expose the superior deep cervical and submandibular lymph nodes. For added exposure the cervical incision can be extended into the contralateral supraclavicular space; this may obviate the need for a counterincision. There is usually no need to excise the submental nodes.

The operation begins with the dissection of the contralateral thyroid lobe with all the accessible nodes, but preservation of the parathyroids. The strap muscles on the ipsilateral side are included in the specimen. The operation proceeds with the dissection of the ipsilateral lobe. The parathyroids are either preserved in situ or transplanted as described on page 102 (Plate 22, B). At this point, the sternocleidomastoid muscle is separated from its sternal and clavicular insertions and the external jugular vein is divided between ligatures **(D)**. The omohyoid muscle is divided to expose the supraclavicular lymph nodes **(E)**.

[Total thyroidectomy with neck dissection *continued on page 108.*]

PLATE 23

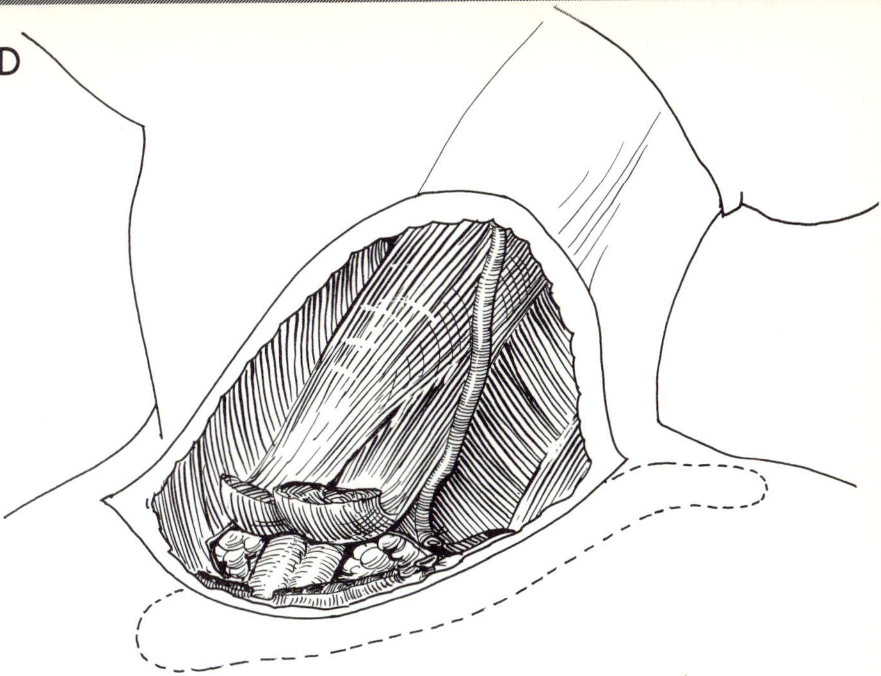

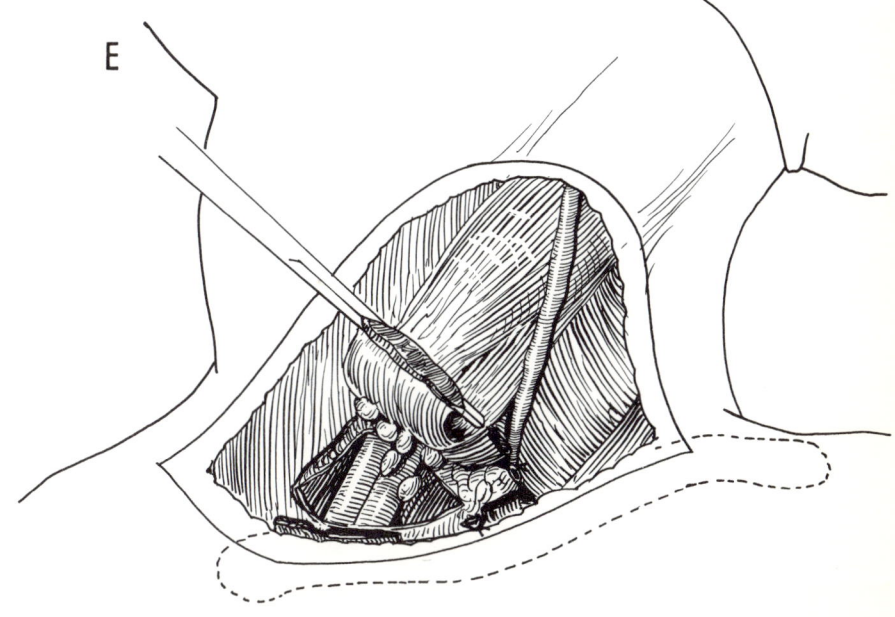

Total Thyroidectomy with Neck Dissection

The internal jugular vein is dissected and divided; its proximal end is doubly ligated with suture ligatures **(F)**.

The following groups of lymph nodes are excised: superior-anterior mediastinal, supraclavicular, inferior deep cervical, transverse cervical, jugulo-omohyoid, external jugular, jugulodigastric, superior deep cervical, submandibular, anterior jugular, infrahyoid and posteriorly the nodes along the course of the accessory nerve. The paratracheal nodes, posterior to the thyroid in the tracheoesophageal groove, are also excised.

To accomplish the desired dissection the sternocleidomastoid muscle must be elevated and rotated posteriorly and laterally, with preservation of its blood supply and part of its innervation **(G)**.

[Total thyroidectomy with neck dissection *continued on page 110.*]

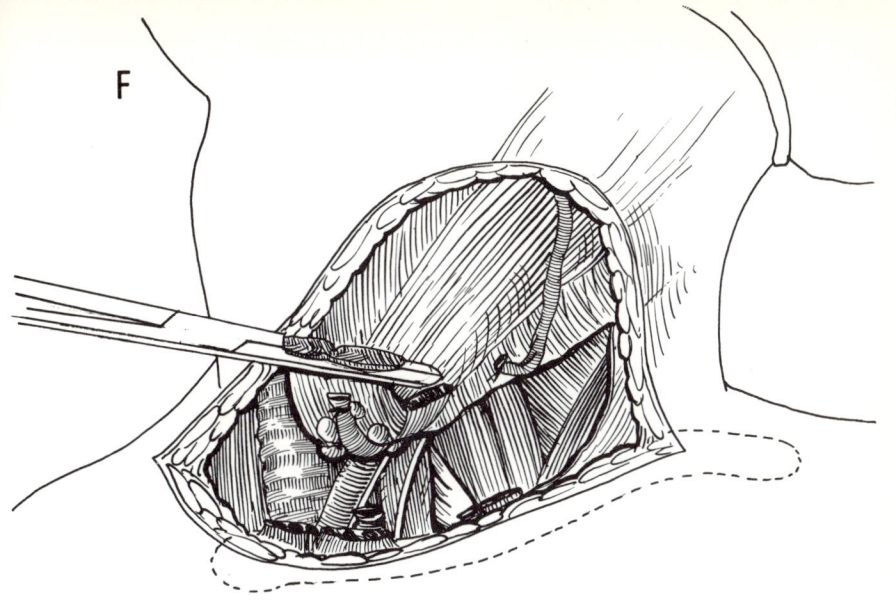

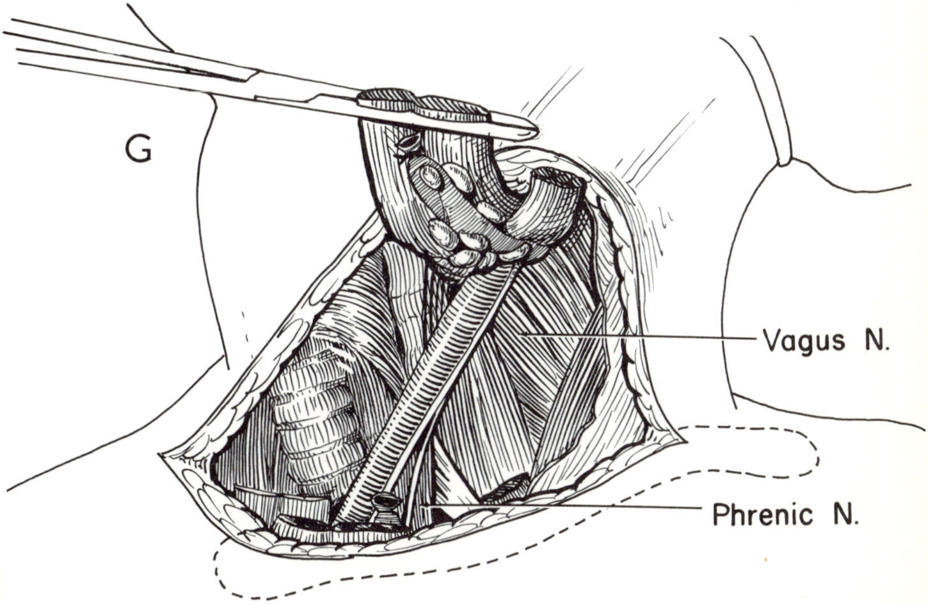

The accessory nerve, the phrenic, vagus, hypoglossal and lingual nerves, the ramus marginalis mandibulae of the facial nerve and, of course, the brachial plexus must be preserved. The supraclavicular, transverse cervical and great auricular nerves can be sacrificed **(H)**. The carotid bulb is infiltrated with a local anesthetic solution during the dissection to avoid bradycardia, vasodilatation and hypotension.

Once the dissection is completed and the various structures that have been preserved identified once more, the sternocleidomastoid muscle is reattached to the clavicle and sternum **(I)**.

[Total thyroidectomy with neck dissection *continued on page 112.*]

PLATE 23

H

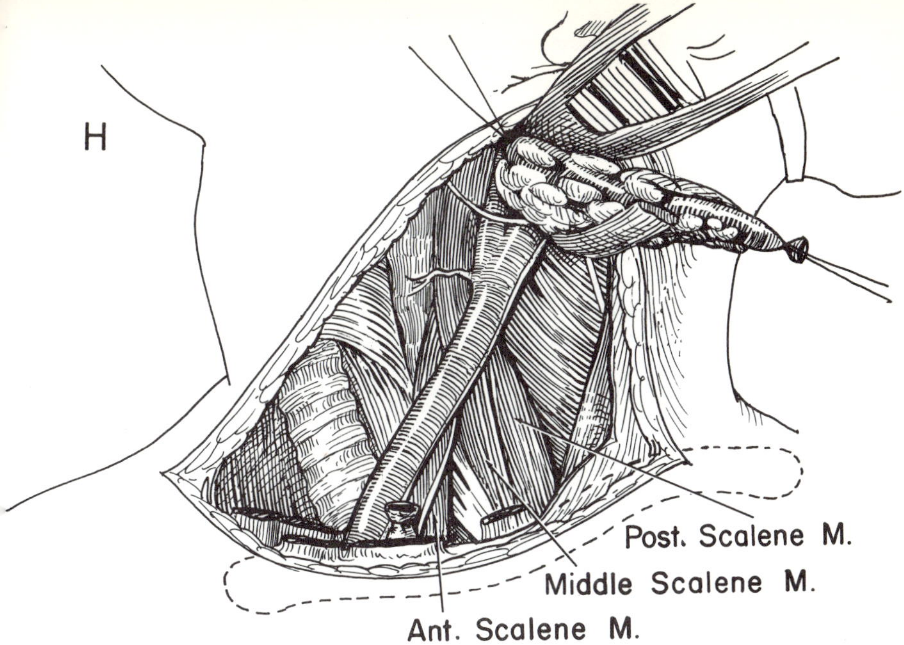
Post. Scalene M.
Middle Scalene M.
Ant. Scalene M.

I

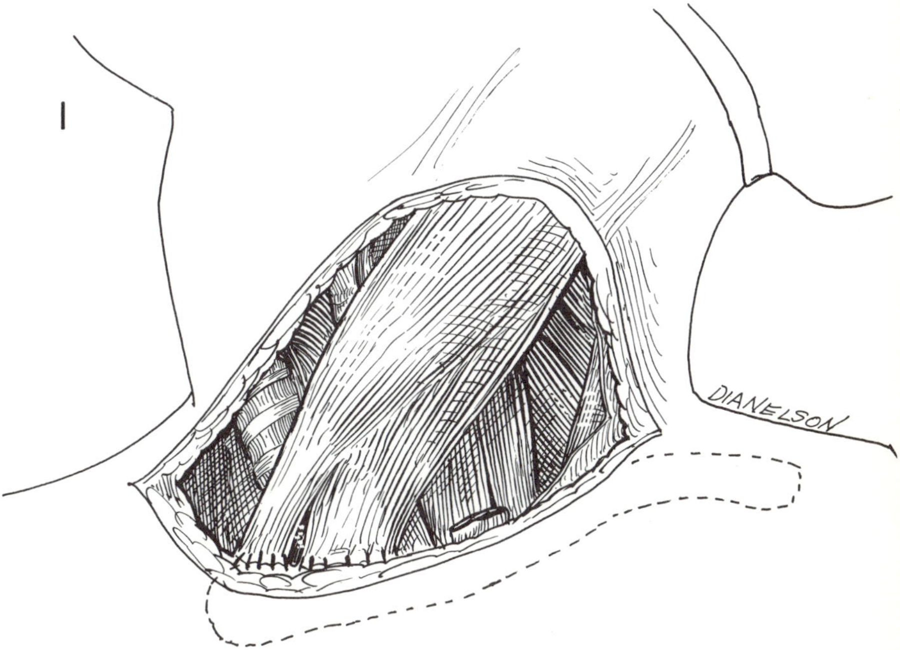
DIANELSON

Subplatysmal space drainage is established with a plastic catheter with multiple perforations, connected to a continuous suction system. The incision is closed **(J)** in the manner described for thyroidectomy (Plate 20). Separate stab wounds lateral to the incision are used for the drainage catheter **(K)**. The catheter is removed within 48 hours.

Even though a total thyroidectomy with a modified neck dissection is a long operation, patients tolerate it quite well and are discharged usually within 4 or 5 days.

In instances of contralateral node involvement, a subsequent modified neck dissection is done some 3–4 months later. The extent of that dissection will be dictated by the findings at operation.

PLATE 23

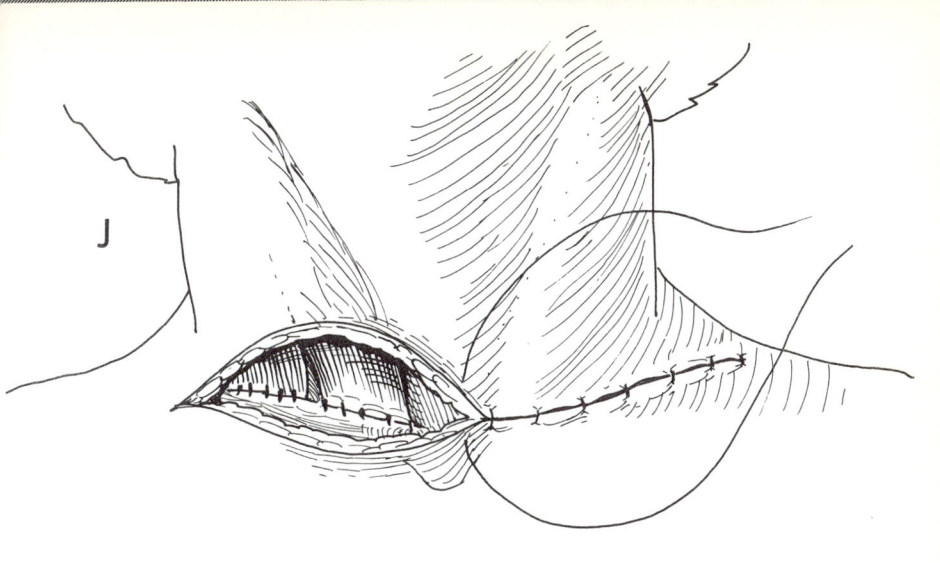

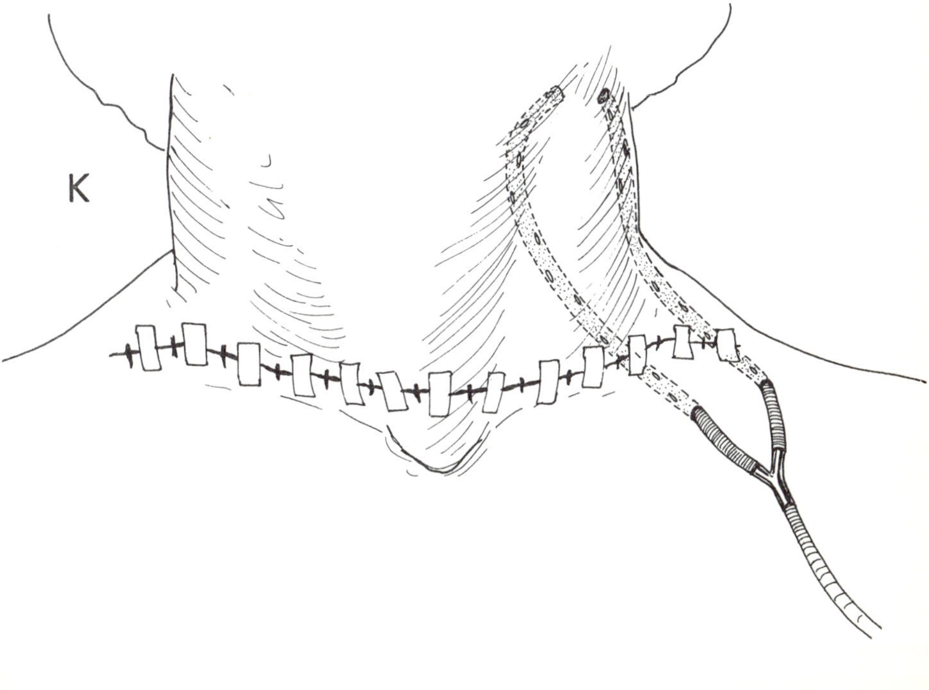

Bilateral Subtotal Resection for Graves' Disease

In contrast to operations for tumors, this is an entirely different physiologic and pathologic situation, which calls for specific preoperative and postoperative considerations and a different operative technic. The most important aspect of the preparation of these patients is the achievement of a euthyroid state (*not* hypothyroid) with a combination of antithyroid drugs and thyroxin. Several weeks to several months may be required to achieve a state where the patient is euthyroid and the gland has undergone involution and developed a firm consistency.

The thyroid gland of a patient with untreated Graves' disease is usually enlarged, with a high flow rate of blood, which accounts for the thyroid bruit. When thyroid blockers are administered (especially when the patient is allowed to slip into a hyopthyroid state), the gland may enlarge under TSH stimulation, becoming even more vascular. For these reasons, during the treatment and preoperative preparation of a patient with Graves' disease, thyroxin is administered as soon as the patient approaches the euthyroid state and before she becomes hypothyroid. For many years Lugol's iodine was used, in conjunction with thyroid blockers, to block TSH and prevent vascular hypertrophy of the thyroid. Thyroxin achieves the same result, with the added advantage of obviating the possibility of hypothyroidism. Since it is not possible to titrate thyroid blockers, a full blocking dose is prescribed; hypothyroidism and TSH stimulation of the gland are prevented by the administration of thyroxin.

Bilateral Subtotal Thyroidectomy [115]

The aim of the surgeon in this operation is to resect the right amount of thyroid tissue. The experience and judgment of the surgeon will define the "right amount." Ideally, such an operation should have a very low complication rate and a recurrence rate of less than 5%. The incidence of long-term hypothyroidism following subtotal thyroidectomy ranges between 20 and 40%. The long-term rate in patients treated with ^{131}I surpasses 80%. Although the incidence of long-term hypothyroidism is related to the coexistence of chronic thyroiditis, which destroys the gland progressively, it may well be that ^{131}I, by an unknown mechanism, accelerates the pre-existing chronic inflammatory process or causes a radiation fibrosis unrelated to it.

During the positioning of the patient on the operating table, special care should be taken to protect the eyes, since many of these patients have exophthalmos. This can be done with an antibiotic ointment and eye pads. The initial steps are similar to those described earlier. The skin incision should be of sufficient length to avoid undue traction and stretching of the skin, since these patients have a propensity to develop hypertrophic scars.

[Technic of bilateral subtotal thyroidectomy *on page 116.*]

The superior pole vessels, the middle thyroid veins and the large branches of the thyroidea ima are divided between ligatures **(A** and **B)**. The pyramidal lobe is dissected and a space is created between the trachea and the isthmus **(C)**, through which a Penrose drain is passed for traction on the isthmus. There is no need (and it is probably unwise) to dissect and locate the recurrent nerves and the parathyroids of these patients, since the line of resection will be some distance from these structures. With the vascularity, edema and lymphatic hyperplasia that exist in the necks of these patients, these structures are difficult to locate and subject to injury.

With all major vessels except the inferior thyroid vessels ligated, the line of resection is demarcated by placing curved hemostats (the points facing upward), *in* the substance of the thyroid **(D)**. With sharp dissection the gland is excised en bloc, except for a 2–3-gm segment of the inferior pole on each side, left attached to the posterior capsule **(E)**. The trachea is completely exposed. Bleeding sites are suture-ligated. It is preferable to leave a greater amount of thyroid tissue than required until all the bleeding is controlled. At that point the remnants can be trimmed to achieve the desired size. The remnants should probably be larger (3–5 gm) in patients with the milder form of the disease, especially when the gland is firm prior to treatment, with the assumption of the coexistence of Hashimoto's thyroiditis, a process which will continue to destroy the gland.

After complete hemostasis has been achieved, drainage is established with a soft rubber drain. The strap muscles are approximated, but *not* too tightly. This will allow escape of fluid from that tight compartment if the drain fails to function adequately. The incision is closed. A nonconstricting, very light dressing is applied. The neck of the patient should be in full view of the hospital staff at all times during the first 24 hours.

PLATE 24

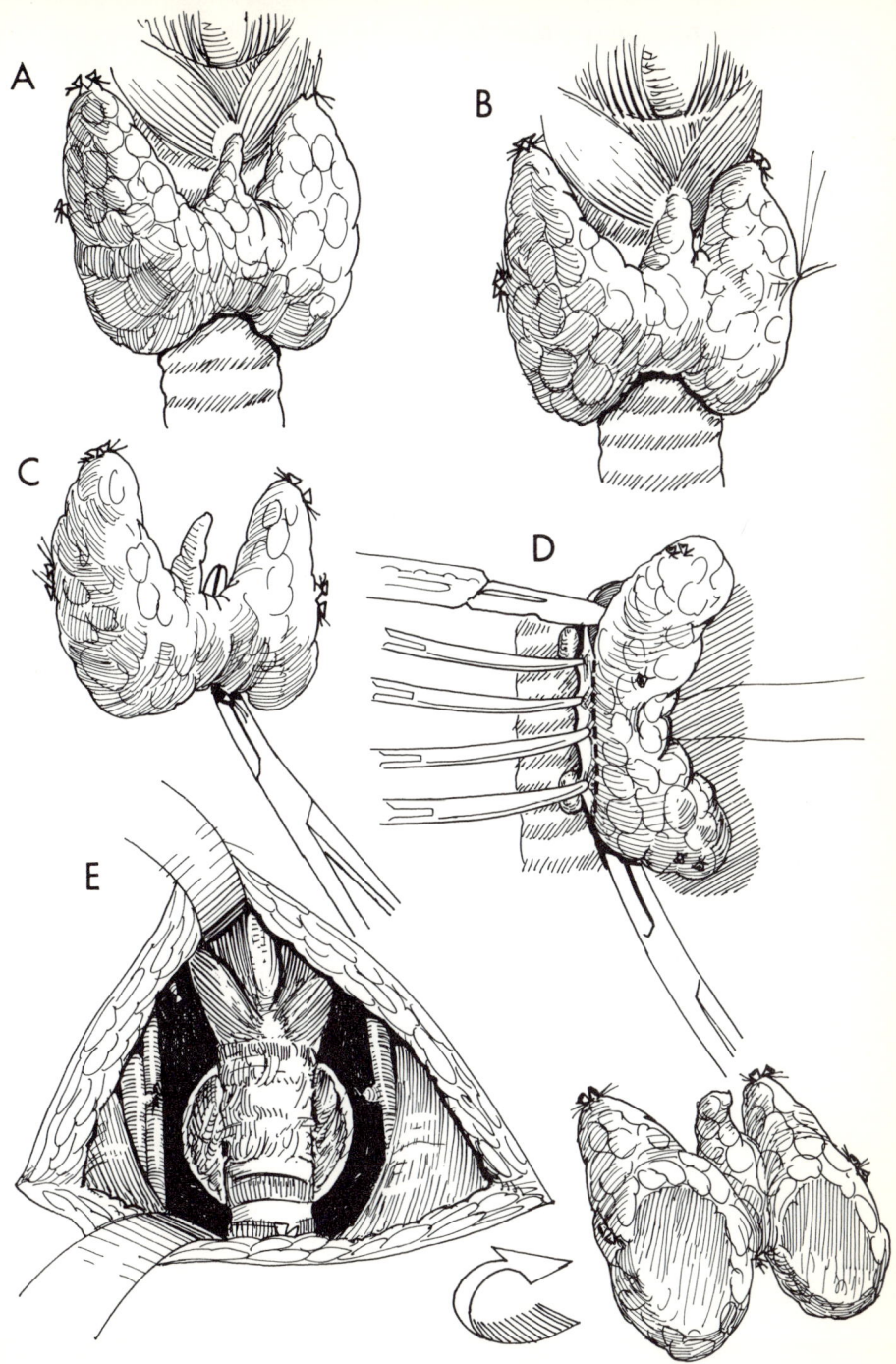

Thyroglossal Duct Cyst Excision

The excision of a thyroglossal duct cyst **(A)** or benign tumor is a rather simple procedure. A transverse submental incision **(B)** will give adequate exposure. The cyst is usually adherent to the thyrohyoid muscle; a few fibers of this muscle are usually part of the surgical specimen. To assure complete excision, with all the sinuses which penetrate in many directions, and to avoid contamination, the cyst should be excised intact, en bloc with all its ramifications **(C)**. Excision of the central portion of the hyoid bone is usually required to obtain better exposure and complete excision **(D and E)**. In some instances the foramen caecum is also excised. The incision is closed primarily after the insertion of a soft rubber drain.

Rare instances of carcinomas arising in thyroglossal duct cysts have been described. These are papillary carcinomas for the most part. The prognosis is excellent, provided a wide excision is done along with bilateral staged neck dissections, which include the submental nodes, when indicated.

PLATE 25

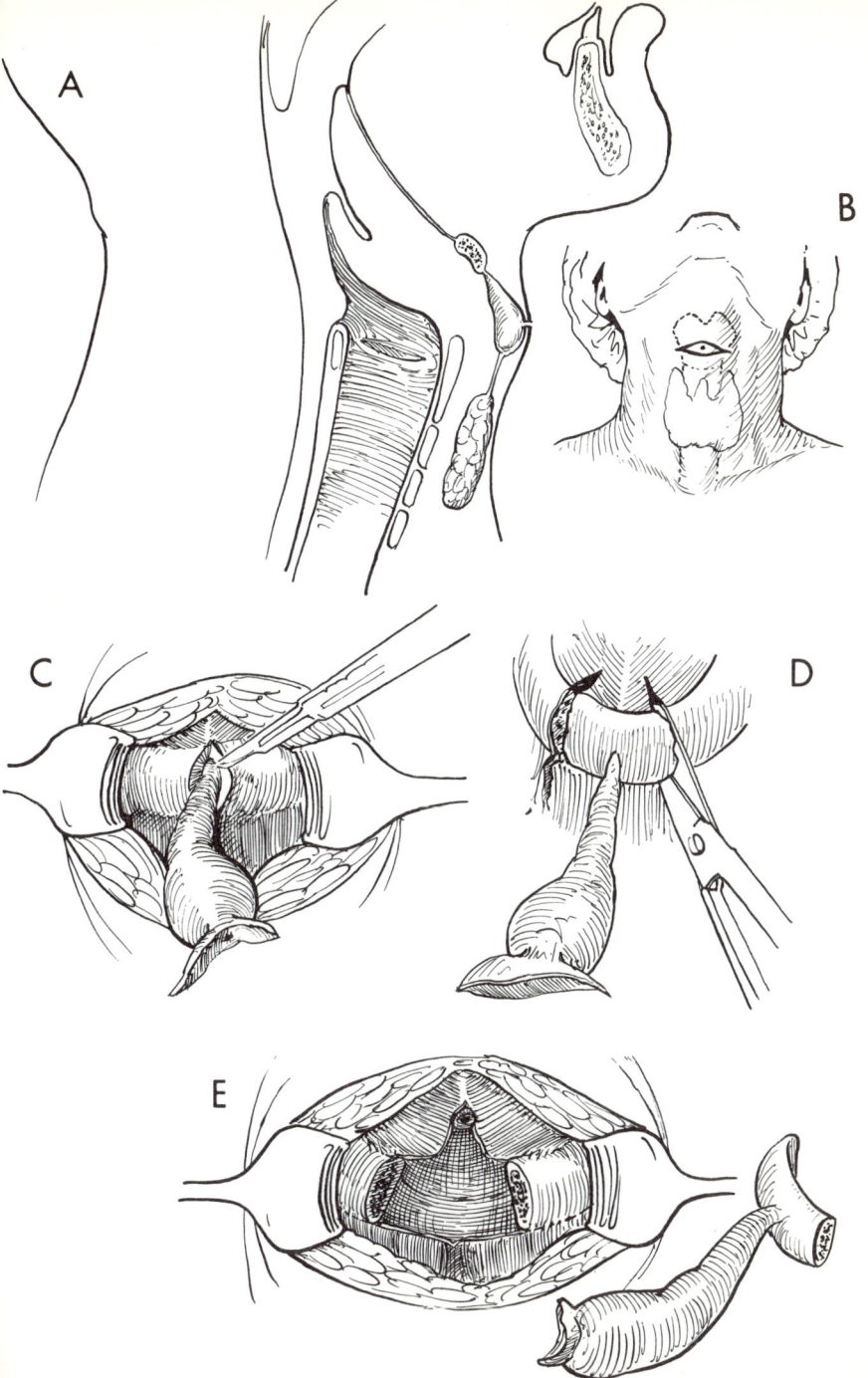

Lingual Thyroid Excision

Undescended thyroid glands are rare; most of them are detected in childhood. They function marginally, and therefore they hypertrophy under TSH stimulation and produce local symptoms. This prolonged TSH stimulation may explain the high (4–6%) incidence of malignancy in lingual thyroids.

Among 400 reported cases of undescended thyroids, 90% were located at the base of the tongue; 10% were in the anterior neck superficial to the hyoid bone.

The diagnosis of undescended thyroid is established by scintigraphy, which confirms also the absence of other thyroid tissue. The treatment of lingual thyroid is TSH suppression with appropriate doses of thyroxin. If this does not produce involution and relief of symptoms, excision is indicated. The simplest approach is by the oral route; exposure is obtained by placing forward traction on the tongue. Complete hemostasis is mandatory; tracheostomy is indicated in most instances. In large tumors, especially if malignancy is suspected, a combination of the oral route and submental transhyoid approach is desirable. In case of malignancy, the appropriate modified neck dissection, which includes a submental node dissection, is done when nodal metastases are demonstrated or when there is marked adenopathy.

In benign cases of lingual thyroid, instances of excision with successful autogenous transplantation have been reported. The value of autogenous transplantation is questionable, since these glands function marginally to begin with. All patients with lingual thyroids should remain on thyroxin permanently, *especially* after excision.

Complications in Thyroid Operations

INTRAOPERATIVE COMPLICATIONS

BLEEDING.—Excessive bleeding at the time of resection should be controlled first with pressure. Then the bleeding points should be precisely identified, with further dissection if necessary, and suture-ligated. Hurried use of hemostats or suture-ligatures may produce injuries to laryngeal nerves or parathyroids.

AIR EMBOLISM.—Large veins in the neck may not bleed even when completely transected. The close proximity to the thoracic outlet and the negative intrathoracic pressure produced by inspiration are factors conducive to air embolism. The best approach is prophylaxis: controlled inhalation with positive pressure at all times, combined with careful and painstaking dissection and hemostasis.

SEVERED RECURRENT NERVE. — If a recurrent nerve is severed, the 2 ends should be reapproximated with fine (6–0 or 7–0) sutures. Normal function returns in over 50% of patients within 12–16 months.

PARATHYROID REIMPLANTATION. — If a parathyroid gland is removed along with the thyroid specimen, this gland should be dissected and reimplanted into the ipsilateral sternocleidomastoid muscle after it has been fragmented into small segments, provided it is not immediately adjacent to a malignant neoplasm. The site of autotransplantation is marked with a metallic clip for future identification.

POSTOPERATIVE COMPLICATIONS

AIRWAY OBSTRUCTION. — Airway obstruction is the most serious complication that may occur during the first 12–24 hours. The combination of endotracheal intubation, dissection of the thyroid gland and manipulation of the larynx leads to substantial laryngeal edema. A minimal amount of bleeding compounds the problem. The combined use of the endotracheal tube and esophageal stethoscope, both rigid structures, is contraindicated in a neck operation where the trachea and larynx are continually manipulated. The esophageal stethoscope should not be utilized in neck operations.

It is preferable to schedule thyroid operations in the morning; thus the patients are fully awake and mobile by evening and capable of alerting the nursing staff if breathing difficulties occur. A tracheostomy set is kept in the patient's room during the first 24 hours for the main purpose of providing the instruments necessary to open the wound and decompress the trachea in case of bleeding. Once this is accomplished, there is usually sufficient time to return the patient to the operating room for the tracheostomy.

In case of impending airway obstruction, ancillary and delaying procedures should be bypassed in favor of an immediate tracheostomy, preferably done in the operating room. Antibiotics are administered for prophylaxis.

BLEEDING.—Exacting hemostasis is imperative in neck operations. Small amounts of blood (30-50 ml) will produce sufficient irritation, edema and compression to cause airway obstruction. Bleeding is more apt to occur after resections for Graves' disease and after neck dissections. The appearance and size of the neck should be under the constant vigil of the staff during the first 24 hours. Wound dressings should be light or altogether absent to facilitate close observation. An experienced nursing staff is invaluable in averting catastrophes and in detecting incipient problems that may at times escape the unaccustomed eyes of the rotating resident staff.

Postoperative bleeding is managed by re-exploration in the operating room under endotracheal general anesthesia. At the conclusion of such a procedure, tracheostomy is a *must;* if not done, it will almost invariably be required after a few hours, during which time the patient's life is endangered by impending airway obstruction.

THYROID STORM.—This problem is seldom seen in this day and age, when most patients with thyrotoxicosis are treated with ^{131}I and the candidates for resection are usually well prepared. Occasionally a patient allergic to antithyroid drugs will refuse ^{131}I therapy; a short course of β-adrenergic blockers (propanolol) and Lugol's iodine is sufficient to avert a thyroid storm.

In the event of storm, treatment consists of any one or a combination of the following measures, beginning with the simplest ones: hydration, Lugol's iodine, propanolol, cooling, antithyroid drugs (unless patient is allergic) and finally hydrocortisone. In a severe crisis it is best to use all of these methods simultaneously.

HYPOCALCEMIA.—Following subtotal thyroidectomy for Graves' disease, in which the inferior posterior portions of each thyroid lobe have not been dissected, hypocalcemia is due to the rapid accretion of calcium back into bone, since many patients with Graves' disease are osteoporotic. The serum phosphorus level is usually normal or low. Parathyroid function is normal. These patients respond well to dietary calcium supplements in the form of milk or calcium lactate wafers administered every 6 hours around the clock. Occasionally they will require calciferol in addition to calcium wafers, to enhance calcium absorption temporarily.

After total thyroidectomy hypocalcemia, with hyperphosphatemia, is the result of hypoparathyroidism; it may be temporary or permanent. If the pathologist finds 4 parathyroid glands on the specimen, the patient is begun on calciferol, dihydrotachysterol and oral calcium gluconate (4 gm every 6 hours) simultaneously, as soon as hypocalcemia and hyperphosphatemia are documented. Dihydrotachysterol is effective within a few hours; after an initial dose of 0.5 mg, 0.375 mg is administered every 6 hours; it is discontinued after approximately 10 days when calciferol, at a dose of 100,000 units daily, reaches full effectiveness. During the ensuing few weeks and months the dose of calciferol is adjusted. Calcium gluconate wafers are discontinued within a few weeks. Rarely, during the first few postoperative days the patient may not tolerate the symptoms of hypocalcemia. Symptomatic relief can be obtained quickly by the very slow intravenous administration of calcium gluconate. The use of undiluted calcium chloride should be avoided, since it is very irritating to the tissues. With such management, temporary or permanent hypoparathyroidism should not delay the patient's discharge from the hospital.

If the parathyroids have been transplanted or there is reason to believe that the patient still possesses some of his or her parathyroids, the regimen described in the preceding paragraph is followed at first. After a few weeks the oral calcium supplements are discontinued. Subsequently, calciferol dosage is gradually reduced and finally discontinued over a period of several weeks. Serum calcium and phosphorus levels will remain normal in over 95% of patients with retained parathyroids. It is noteworthy that, when such patients are rendered hypothyroid by withdrawal of thyroxin therapy in preparation for postoperative ^{131}I scanning, hypocalcemia and mild symptoms may develop. This is invariably corrected by the resumption of thyroxin therapy.

CORNEAL ABRASION. — This tends to occur in patients with exophthalmos when the eyes are not well protected during operation. It is treated with antibiotic ophthalmic drops administered every 2 hours and an eye patch. The lesion heals rapidly without sequelae. The symptoms subside within 24 hours.

RECURRENT NERVE PALSY. — Injury to the recurrent nerve(s) is a constant danger in all thyroid resections from the time the gland is exposed until the strap muscles are approximated. Situations in which the recurrent nerve must be sacrificed to obtain complete resection of a tumor are rare indeed.

The first clue of a recurrent nerve injury is the inability of the patient to cough in the recovery room. Inability to project the voice and to phonate high-pitched tones will be noted subsequently. Occasionally recurrent nerve palsy will occur during the postoperative period, even though it may have been absent in the recovery room or on the first postoperative day. This is probably due to edema and compression; the chances of recovery are excellent.

Before discharge the function of the vocal cords should be examined by means of indirect laryngoscopy by an independent observer in all patients who have undergone a thyroidectomy.

In instances of documented recurrent nerve palsy, the patient is instructed in the performance of exercises to develop compensation for the paralyzed vocal cord. The contralateral vocal cord may cross the midline and compensate to such a degree that the voice may become almost normal. In patients in whom the vocal cord remains paralyzed after 18 months and who are unable to phonate to their satisfaction, the injection of Teflon will impart some rigidity to the affected cord and restore excellent approximation and function.

In bilateral cord paralysis a tracheostomy may be required. One of the cords may have to be injected with Teflon or just glycerin if there is no return of function after a suitable period of time.

SUPERIOR LARYNGEAL NERVE PALSY. — Injury to this nerve produces no noticeable impairment unless the patient is a singer or has to speak for long periods. Most patients will compensate for this after a few months. However, singers will continue to have difficulty in reaching high-pitched tones.

KELOIDS. — This unsightly complication is more apt to occur in patients operated on for Graves' disease and in the black population. Keloids can be treated and reduced to flat, broad scars with applications or local injections of triamcinolone.

ASYMMETRIC SCAR. — Asymmetry may occur following the excision of large nodules; the best therapy is prophylaxis. This complication is prevented by judicious planning of the incision: the incision on the side of a large nodule should be lower (closer to the clavicle) than on the contralateral side. The degree of dissymmetry in the planning of the incision is proportional to the size of the nodule.

Postoperative Management

THYROTOXIC STATES. — Patients operated on for Graves' disease or other toxic states should require no medication postoperatively. Serum thyroxin levels should be determined monthly during the first 3 months and yearly therafter. Some patients with Graves' disease may become hypothyroid after many years. This is probably due to the destruction of thyroid parenchyma by chronic thyroiditis.

In case of recurrence of hyperthyroidism, ^{131}I therapy is the treatment of choice. A few patients with long-standing Graves' disease will become hypocalcemic after resection. This phenomenon is usually not due to hypoparathyroidism, but rather to the rapid accretion of calcium into the skeleton, which has been depleted over a long period of time; it is another form of bone hunger. Serum phosphorus levels are usually low or normal. This hypocalcemia is treated with calciferol and oral calcium supplements until the symptoms have subsided (see the section on Hypocalcemia).

BENIGN AND MALIGNANT TUMORS. — There is ample evidence that TSH stimulates growth and hyperplasia of thyroid parenchyma; in animal models this leads to metastasizing tumors, which regress completely with TSH suppression. Following thyroidectomy for benign tumors, replacement doses of thyroxine are prescribed. Patients with malignancies are treated with larger suppressive doses. The efficacy of treatment can be ascertained with circulating thyroxin and TSH measurements.

Patients with residual uptake of ^{131}I of the thyroid bed or other locations after an operation for thyroid cancer are treated with large doses of ^{131}I after a hypothyroid state has been induced. Then suppressive doses of thyroxin are resumed. The patient is scanned again a few months later; ^{131}I is administered again if any significant uptake is noted. Female patients should avoid pregnancy during this phase of treatment, since the fetal thyroid starts functioning during the twelfth to the fourteenth week of pregnancy.

CHAPTER 3

Islet Cell Tumors of the Pancreas

The adult human pancreas weighs 50–70 gm. The islets weigh a total of approximately 1 gm; their size ranges from 20 to 300 μ in diameter. The total number varies between 1 and 2 million; in other words, the average weight of each islet is less than 1 μg. The islets are composed of 4 cell types: the alpha cells, which secrete glucagon; the beta cells, which are the seat of insulin synthesis; the D cells, which secrete gastrin in all probability, and the agranular C cells, of unknown function. In the human pancreas 60–80% of the islet cells are of the beta variety.

Historical Highlights

The history of the study of the islets of Langerhans and their secretions is embroidered with a series of fundamental discoveries that have provided a blueprint for the study of other endocrine glands.

MORPHOLOGIC HISTORY

Langerhans, while still a medical student in 1869, discovered and described the islets, which Laguesse subsequently named after their discoverer. In 1882 Kuhe and Lea described the capillary network in which the islet cells are embedded. Then, in 1886, Lewaschew reported a very scholarly study in which he demonstrated the stimulation of insular growth by overfeeding or by pilocarpine administration.

In 1893 Laguesse described the histology, including the granules, of the islets and their capillary network and suggested, purely on morphologic grounds, that they were organs of internal secretion.

The next histologic advance came in 1906 when Lane reported his famous staining technic, by which he demonstrated 2 types of granules in the islets; he called them alpha and beta. In 1912 Bensley added a vital staining method to the technical procedure; this enabled him to demonstrate the origin of both types of cells from ductular epithelium in contradistinction to acinar elements and to count the number of islets in the adult guinea pig, which he estimated at 56,000, vastly more than the opponents of the endocrine school had claimed. Bensley also described the third, nongranular C cell.

In 1924 Bowie described alpha, beta and gamma granular cells in teleost fish, and in 1931 Bloom described the same cells in man.

Metabolic History

The history of the relationship of the islets of Langerhans to clinical metabolic problems had its inception as far back as 1788, when Cawley described the finding of pancreatic calculi in a patient with diabetes mellitus. This marked the beginning of the concept, which developed over the next hundred years, that the pancreas might be implicated in diabetes.

In 1849 Claude Bernard published his famous monograph, in which he describes his discovery of hyperglycemia and glycosuria in diabetes. In 1889 Mering and Minkowski observed that many features of clinical diabetes were reproduced in experimental animals by pancreatectomy.

In 1894 Hedon lent strong support to the theory that diabetes is caused by a defect in pancreatic endocrine secretion when he showed that the development of clinical diabetes could be prevented by transplanting a portion of the pancreas devoid of neural connections into the subcutaneous tissues.

In 1909 Meyer was so confident that the pancreas secreted a substance capable of supporting life in the absence of the organ itself that he coined the word "insuline" to designate this substance despite the many unfruitful attempts to extract it. This failure of extraction attempts was attributed to the hydrolyzation of insulin by the proteolytic enzymes secreted by the acinar tissue.

In 1922 the problem of proteolytic enzyme contamination was circumvented by Banting and Best, who ligated the ducts of the pancreas and allowed degeneration of the acinar tissue prior to their successful extraction of insulin from the intact islets. This has been considered the most significant event in this series of discoveries, despite the fact that it constitutes merely a technical feat.

In 1926 Abel was able to purify insulin by crystallization and estimated its molecular weight at 34,500. Crystalline insulin did not produce the initial hyperglycemic effect that had been noted with the administration of impure extracts. The absence of this hyperglycemic effect was the first clue that the impure extracts contained a glycolytic substance, later to be identified as glucagon.

In 1954 Sanger and Tuppy determined the amino acid sequence of insulin.

In 1960 another milestone was erected when Berson and Yallow reported a highly sensitive immunoassay for insulin, a methodology that has since been applied to many other hormones and has revolutionized the world of endocrinology.

In 1967 Steiner, in a study of the biosynthesis of insulin in beta cell tumor tissue slices, discovered an insulin precursor that he named proinsulin. This set the stage for the isolation and characterization of other prohormones.

The history of glucagon is less dramatic and shorter. A clue to its existence was the initial hyperglycemic effect of the first impure extracts of pancreatic islets for insulin. When this hyperglycemic effect was eliminated by the purification and crystallization of insulin, the stage was set for the discovery of glucagon. As early as 1930 this hypothetical substance was named glucagon. In 1948 the glycogenolytic effect of glucagon in liver slices was demonstrated by Cori and by Heard and his associates. Five years later Staub was able to purify glucagon, and 2 years later, in 1954, Bromer and Behrens crystallized glucagon and determined its amino acid sequence. During the late 1960s and early 1970s glucagon research fell into a state of relative inanition, until glucagon became the subject of a dramatic revival when its role in the ketogenesis of diabetes was appreciated.

Since the discovery of the Zollinger-Ellison gastrin-secreting tumors in 1955, followed by extensive morphologic and biochemical studies of these tumors and of the islets of Langerhans, 2 varieties of alpha cells and 2 other cells have been described: the D cells, which are thought to secrete gastrin, and the C cells, which have an unknown function.

History of Islet Cell Tumors

In 1902 Nicholls, a pathologist, recorded the first islet cell tumor. Other sporadic reports followed. These tumors were to be regarded as pathologic curiosities with no clinical significance during the next quarter of a century.

In 1908 Seale Harris first described the concept of organic hyperinsulinism and thus paved the way for Wilder and co-workers, who in 1927 established the unquestionable correlation between clinical hyperinsulinism and a malignant islet cell tumor they found at operation. In 1929 Roscoe Graham was the first to report a case of operative cure of organic hyperinsulinism. By 1950 almost 400 cases had been collected in the literature, and by 1958 this number was approaching 1,000.

The next milestone occurred in 1955, when Zollinger and Ellison reported their first 2 patients with primary peptic ulceration of the jejunum associated with islet cell tumors (gastrinomas) of the pancreas. Actually, Hilger Perry Jenkins, another surgeon, had called their attention to the possibility of such an association based on his observations in another patient.

In the 1960s other functioning varieties of islet cell tumors were reported. These included glucagonomas and tumors associated with the syndrome of watery diarrhea, hypokalemia and achlorhydria or hypochlorhydria (WDHA). Furthermore, these islet cell tumors are capable of synthesizing and secreting a variety of nonpancreatic hormones, such as calcitonin, PTH, melanocyte-stimulating hormone (MSH), adrenocorticotropic hormone (ACTH), serotonin and other hormones of enteric and nonenteric origin. Finally in the 1970s the WDHA syndrome was characterized as a distinct syndrome associated with "non-beta" islet cell tumors of the pancreas. Although secretin and a variety of vasoactive intestinal peptides have been suspected, the "diarrheogenic hormone" responsible has defied identification and characterization.

Physiology

To this day, of the 3 known secretions of the islets, only insulin has a well-defined role. An important pathophysiologic role for glucagon is emerging currently.

INSULIN.—A normal adult man secretes approximately 50 units of insulin in 24 hours. The actions of insulin are wide-ranging, with well-defined influences on many organ systems.

Insulin has a primary role in carbohydrate metabolism. Its regulation of the transmission of glucose through a variety of cell walls is merely the first step in a long series of metabolic pathways governed by it.

In lipid metabolism insulin stimulates lipogenesis and lipolysis and reduces the amount of energy derived from fat. The influence of insulin extends to cholesterol synthesis and ketogenesis.

In protein metabolism insulin deficiency leads to decreased protein synthesis and increased gluconeogenesis, with resulting protein catabolism and negative nitrogen balance, which in turn leads to impaired growth in young subjects and poor healing of wounds in diabetic patients. Impaired mucopolysaccharide synthesis in diabetics undoubtedly contributes to many of the complications seen in this disorder, since acid mucopolysaccharides are a common constituent of connective tissue and are known to exert an important role in wound healing and resistance to infection.

GLUCAGON.—Although the physiologic role of glucagon has not been well defined, many of its metabolic actions have been characterized.

The principal action of glucagon seems to be on the liver, where it stimulates glycogenolysis, gluconeogenesis, lipolysis, ketogenesis and proteolysis. It also produces lipolysis in adipose tissue. One of its most important actions may be its direct stimulatory effect on the release of insulin from beta cells. The highly vascular complex interspersed between the islet cells, the continuous pericapillary spaces, which may help in the distribution of secretions from 1 pancreatic cell to another, and the close juxtaposition of the alpha and beta cells are morphologic observations that emphasize the possibility of an important physiologic role for the highly stimulatory effect of glucagon on insulin secretion. Very recently, the role of glucagon in the development of ketosis in diabetics has been the focus of intensive investigation. This concept has been supported by the dramatic correction of ketosis in diabetics out of control by the mere administration of somatostatin, a hypothalamic polypeptide that inhibits glucagon release.

Although neural control of insular secretion has been suspected since the turn of the century, when neuroinsular complexes were described by histochemists, it was not demonstrated until the early 1970s. Sympathetic nerves and adrenergic substances stimulate glucagon secretion via β-adrenergic receptors. In contrast, adrenergic substances inhibit insulin release via α-receptors.

GASTRIN.—It is only recently that the secretory granules of the D cells have been shown to contain gastrin. The physiologic role of pancreatic gastrin has not been defined.

Histology

Embryologically both the exocrine and endocrine portions of the pancreas are thought to have a common origin from cords of cells growing out of the ducts from the foregut and hepatic diverticulum. The islets seem to lose most of their connections with the duct system after the twelfth week of embryonic life, when insulin synthesis begins. Insulin is demonstrable in the pancreas of the human fetus at the beginning of the fourth month.

However, a new school of though proclaims that a majority of the cells in the foregut endocrine system, which share common cytochemical properties, develop in common from neuroectodermal cells that have migrated from the neural crest. These precursor cells in mouse embryos will develop fluorescence after injection of an exogenous precursor of L-dopa into the pregnant mouse. The migration of the fluorescent neuroepidermal cells from the neural crest to the epithelium of the endoderm of the pharyngeal pouches, stomach, duodenum and pancreas has been demonstrated. These endocrine cells, once totipotential, are located in the human foregut from the anterior pituitary to the mid-duodenum and pancreas and in the adrenal medulla, paraganglionic tissues and other mesodermal areas.

In situations where the growth of islets is stimulated, morphologic studies leave little doubt that new islets arise from pancreatic ducts (nesidioblastosis). How this can be reconciled with the theory of neuroectodermal origin of human foregut endocrine cells remains an enigma.

In a normal man the islets are composed of 3 types of granular cells, alpha, beta and delta. The C cells are agranular. All these cells have characteristic morphologic features that can be distinguished with specific histochemical technics, by light microscopy and by electron microscopy.

The fine structure of the beta cells varies from species to species, but the alpha cells have a relatively uniform appearance. Nerve fibers and their terminations on islet cells, which were described at the turn of the century, have received greater attention in recent years with the documentation of the influence of the sympathetic nerve on the secretions of the islets. Electron microscopy has shown that these nerve endings closely applied to plasma membranes of islet cells are unmyelinated.

Finally, the size and the number of the islets increases as one proceeds from the head toward the tail of the pancreas. It is of interest that in the dog's uncinate process, derived from the ventral pancreas, the islets are composed of beta cells and devoid of alpha cells, whereas in the body and the tail, derived from the dorsal pancreas, the islets contain both the alpha and beta varieties.

PLATE 26

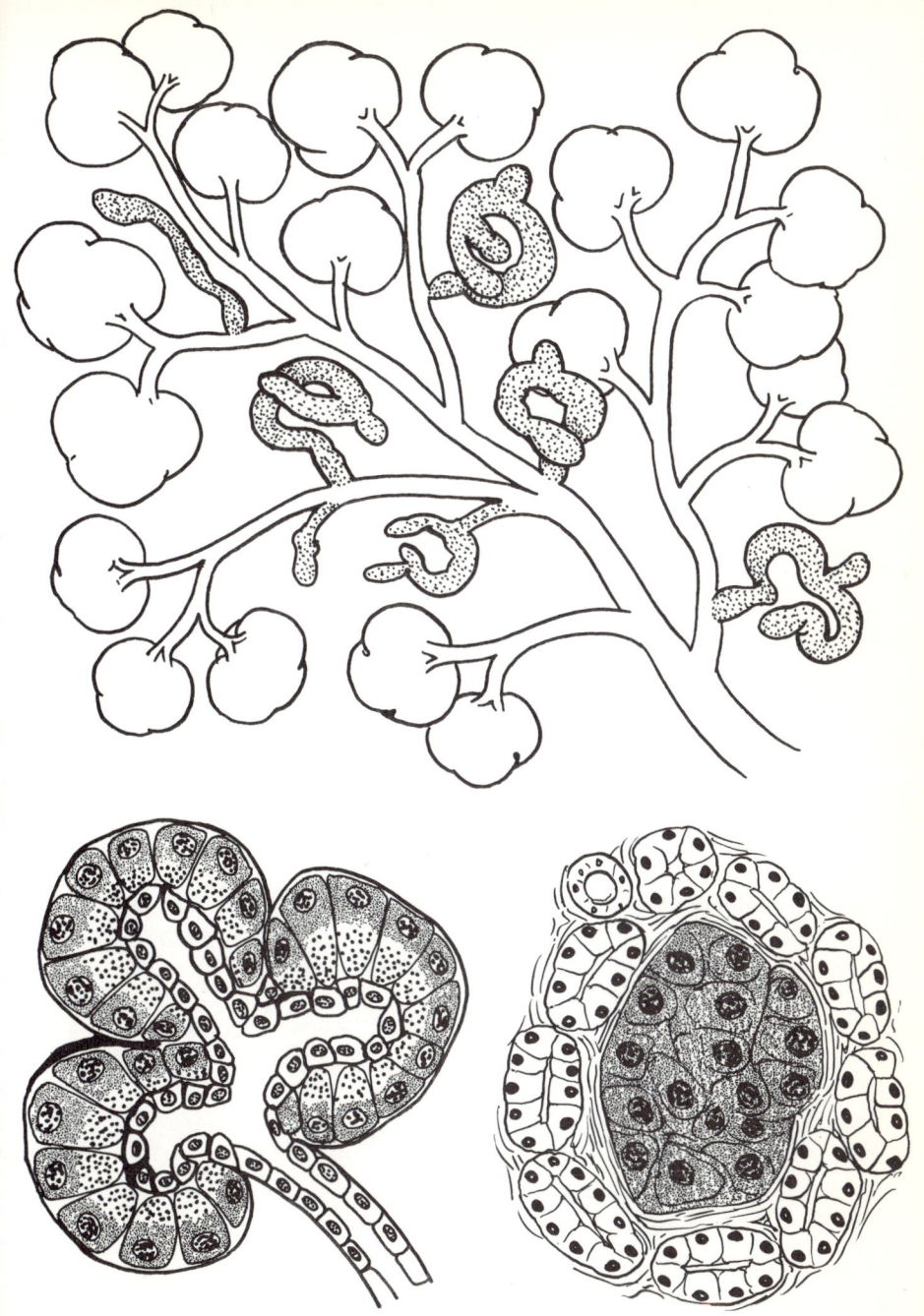

Islet Cell Tumors

Islet cell tumors and the hormones they elaborate are an excellent example of the multiple endocrine adenomatosis syndrome (MEA) and substantiate the concept of the neuroectodermal origin of the peptide-secreting endocrine glands and the unified concept for the etiology of multiple endocrine adenomatosis.

CLASSIFICATION.—Islet cell tumors can best be classified by a combination of cell types and clinical syndromes:

Cell Type	Secretion	Syndrome
Alpha	Glucagon	Hyperglycemia
Beta	Insulin	Hypoglycemia
Delta	Gastrin	Zollinger-Ellison
Non-beta	?	WDHA
Non-beta	Multiple hormones	Mixed endocrinopathy

The "non-beta" tumors, which produce a clinical picture of mixed endocrinopathy, secrete a variety of hormones, including secretin, ACTH, PTH, serotonin, antidiuretic hormone (ADH), MSH and catecholamines.

SIZE AND LOCATION.—The diameter of islet cell tumors is seldom greater than several centimeters. In large series the average size is approximately 1.5–2 cm. They occur throughout the pancreas **(A)**, with the highest incidence in the head (25%) and the tail (35%). They may occur as single tumors or in association with multiple microadenomas **(B)**.

As many as 60% of these tumors can be malignant. Metastases will occur in the abdomen throughout the peritoneal cavity, in the liver, in many groups of lymph nodes, along the gastrointestinal tract, in the kidneys, the lungs, the pleura, the pericardium, the bone marrow and the thyroid. A significant number of these metastases "function" and create severe and lethal metabolic problems secondary to uncontrolled quantities of hormones they secrete.

[Location of islet cell tumors *continued on page 136.*]

PLATE 27

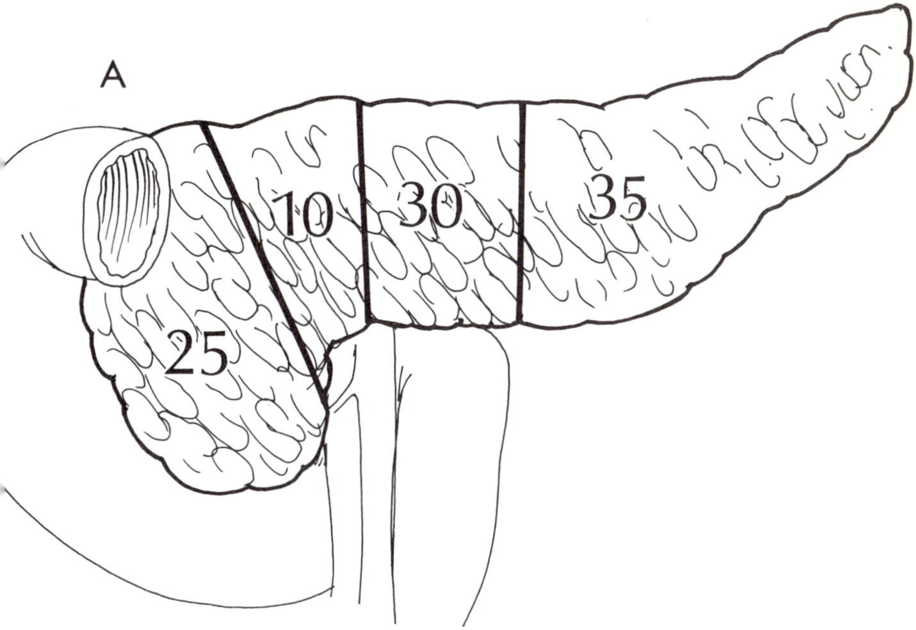

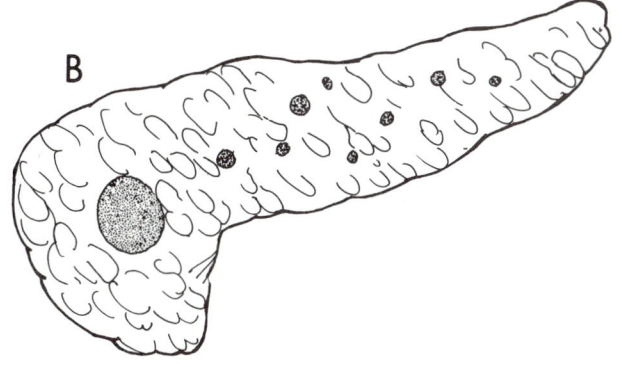

Approximately 3–10% of islet cell tumors are ectopic. Ectopic locations, in decreasing order of frequency, include the duodenum *(2)*, the hilus of the spleen *(4,6,8)*, the retroperitoneum in the vicinity of the pancreas *(3)*, the stomach *(1)*, the biliary tract *(10)* and the bronchi. Rarely they are found in the small bowel *(7,9)* or in a Meckel's diverticulum *(5)*.

HISTOPATHOLOGY. — In general, islet cell tumors are very vascular and can be considered structurally as gigantic islets, faithfully reproducing on a large scale the normal aspects and structural relations of the islets of Langerhans. The normal histologic characteristics are exaggerated and repeated. The general appearance is that of typical or atypical "islet" cells in long or short anastomosing cords, ribbons or strands 1–4 cells in thickness. In the majority the so-called ribbon (trabecular) pattern predominates. In others an alveolar, tubular or rosette arrangement is the rule, and in still others the architecture is that of simple solid tumors. However, these different patterns occur frequently side by side within the same tumor or in the same patient, and therefore classification of cellular patterns seems to serve little purpose. The prevailing characteristic in all these patterns is that of an orderly arrangement of the cells and uniformity in cellular size in a given adenoma.

Thin-walled capillary blood vessels course everywhere among these anastomosing bands of tumor cells except in areas of fibrosis or hyaline change. A delicate fibrous connective tissue framework accompanies the blood vessels and appears condensed in the form of a thin or thick capsule about the periphery of the tumor, where the surrounding pancreatic acinar and duct tissue is frequently compressed.

Under high magnification the individual cells are strikingly similar to those of normal islets. The nuclei are indistinguishable from those of normal insular cells, being small, spherical or ovoid and poor in chromatin. Occasional giant forms are observed. True mitotic figures are uncommon. With special staining technics typical and atypical granulations can be found in the majority of the cells. In most instances the cells will be uniformly of a single variety with either alpha, beta or delta granulations. In patients with mixed endocrinopathies, with the use of more sensitive cytochemical technics, a mixture of these cells will be found. Further, in some of these cellular elements the argentaffin and chromaffin reactions are

PLATE 28

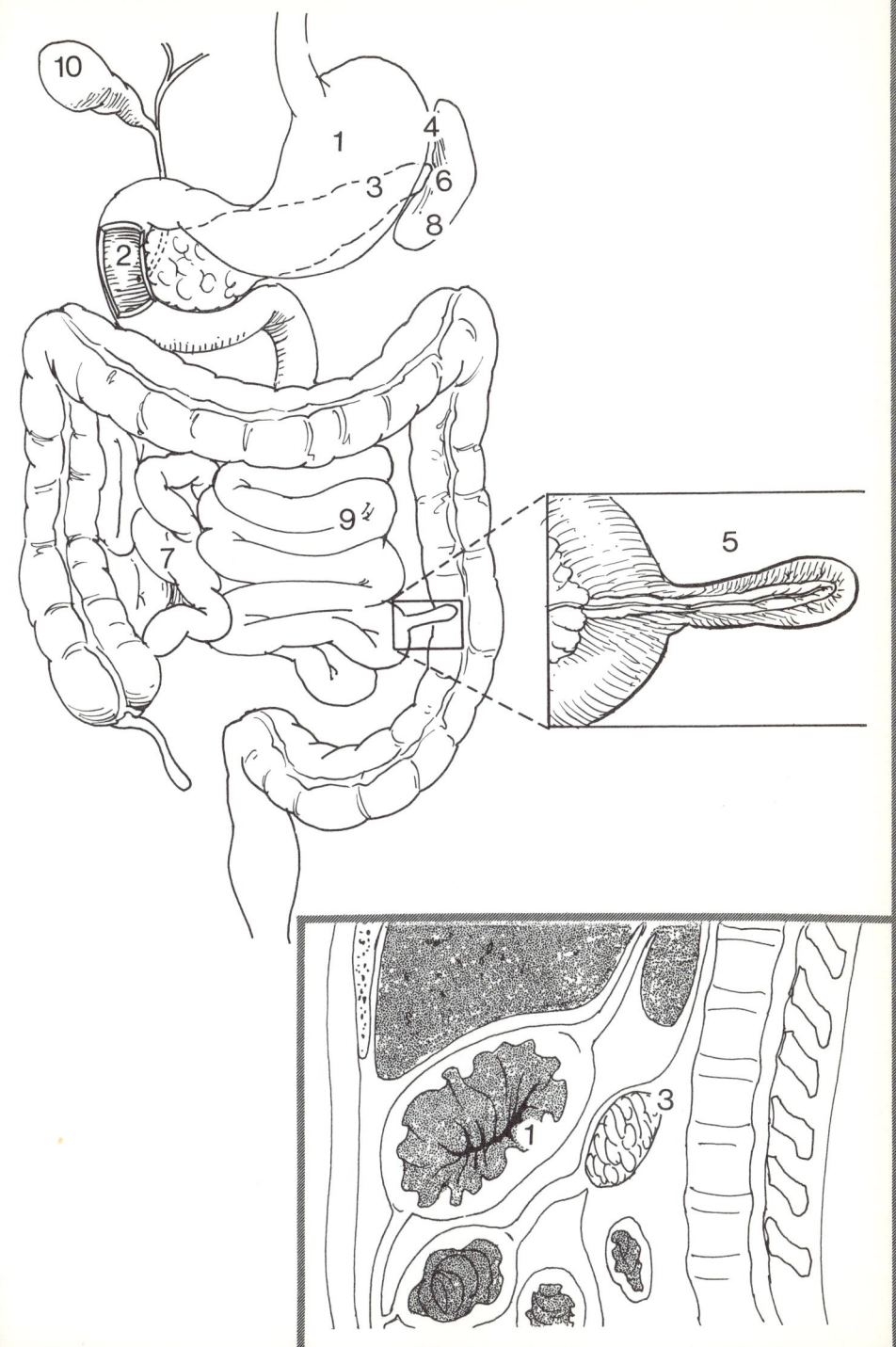

both present in the same cells, a finding suggesting that these cells produce serotonin and catecholamines.

Even though dedifferentiation occurs commonly in the metastases of these tumors, it is surprising to note that the anaplastic cells of the islet cell carcinomas can produce the natural hormones in over half the cases that have been studied. The final characteristic that bears emphasis is that these tumors are slow-growing and produce their deleterious effects principally by the overproduction of natural hormones, even when the growth is widespread and extensive.

Embryology of the Pancreas

The pancreas develops from 2 separate outgrowths of the foregut in the vicinity of the duodenum. In man almost all of the pancreas (tail, body and a portion of the head) is derived from the dorsal pancreas **(A)**. In contrast, the ventral pancreas consists of 2 buds that arise from the hepatic diverticulum and lie on either side of the common bile duct. The left bud usually atrophies. The common bile duct along with the left duct migrate counterclockwise dorsally around the right side of the duodenum **(B)**. This bud forms the remaining segment of the head of the human pancreas.

Each of the 2 pancreatic outgrowths has a single main duct **(C)**; these 2 ducts fuse within the head. The duct of the dorsal pancreas persists as the main duct of the body and tail; in the head it fuses with the main duct of the ventral pancreas, which contributes the terminal portion of the main duct of the pancreas **(D)**. The terminal portion of the duct of the dorsal pancreas usually persists as the accessory duct of Santorini, which enters into the duodenum just proximal to the ampulla of Vater and the duct of Wirsung. The fusion of these 2 ducts accounts for the meandering course of the main pancreatic duct in the head, a characteristic finding in normal pancreatograms **(E)**.

In the dog the ventral pancreas forms the uncinate process, a long segment of pancreatic tissue located along the lesser curvature of the duodenum. In comparison to the islets in the body and tail, the islets of Langerhans in the uncinate process are smaller, fewer and devoid of alpha cells.

PLATE 29

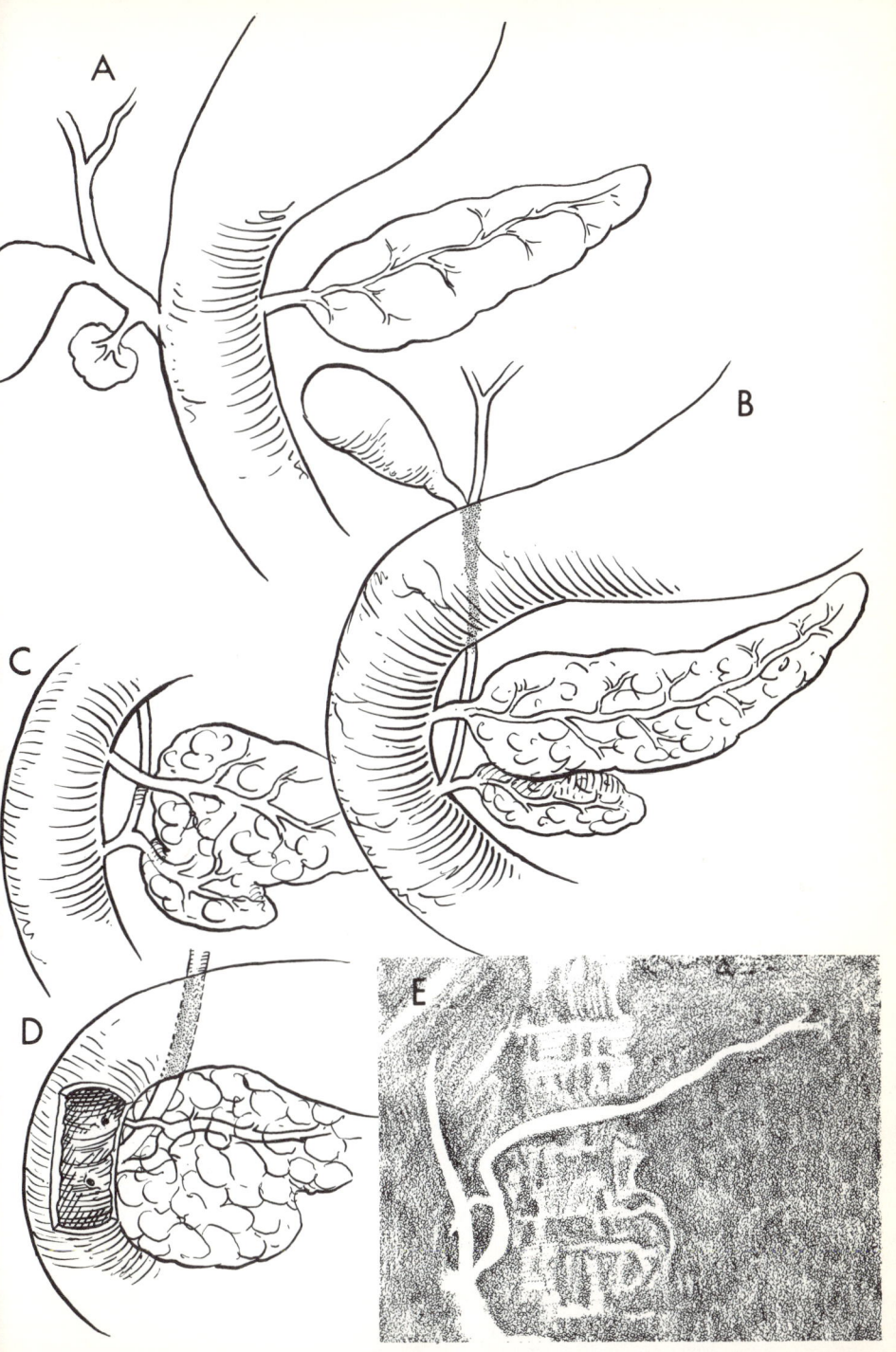

Anatomy of the Pancreas

The pancreas, a pinkish white lobulated structure located in the upper retroperitoneum, extends from the lesser curvature of the duodenum transversely and obliquely across the vena cava and aorta to the hilus of the spleen.

An understanding of the embryonic development of the pancreas is essential to comprehend the anatomy of the gland and its relationship to neighboring structures and organs. As visualized in transverse **(A)** and sagittal **(B)** projections, the ventral and dorsal pancreatic outgrowths arise originally in the biliary and duodenal mesenteries. As these 2 primordia fuse, the dorsal pancreas develops and migrates into the retroperitoneum in such a fashion that its mesentery fuses to the mesentery of the transverse colon. The net result is that, as seen in a sagittal view, the body and tail of the pancreas are located within the retroperitoneum at a point where the 2 peritoneal surfaces of the transverse mesocolon separate **(B, *stage II*)**. Although the head and the body of the pancreas are anterior to the superior mesenteric vessels and the middle colic artery, the uncinate process insinuates itself between the aorta and the superior mesenteric artery. In other words, with its body anterior to the superior mesenteric vessels and its uncinate process posterior to them, the pancreas really forms a collar around the vascular and lymphatic supply to the entire small bowel distal to the duodenum and the ascending and transverse colon. It is small wonder that acute pancreatitis may interfere with the venous and lymphatic drainage of the small bowel and proximal colon. This produces the classic x-ray findings of paralytic ileus, with distention of the small bowel and the ascending and transverse colon. This distention stops abruptly at the splenic flexure; the contrast between the distended transverse colon and its normal descending limb forms the basis for the well-known radiographic splenic flexure cutoff sign.

PLATE 30

B
Spleen
Pancreas
A
A
B

B
STAGE
I
(SAGITTAL)

A
RT.
LT.
(TRANSVERSE)

B
STAGE
II
(SAGITTAL)

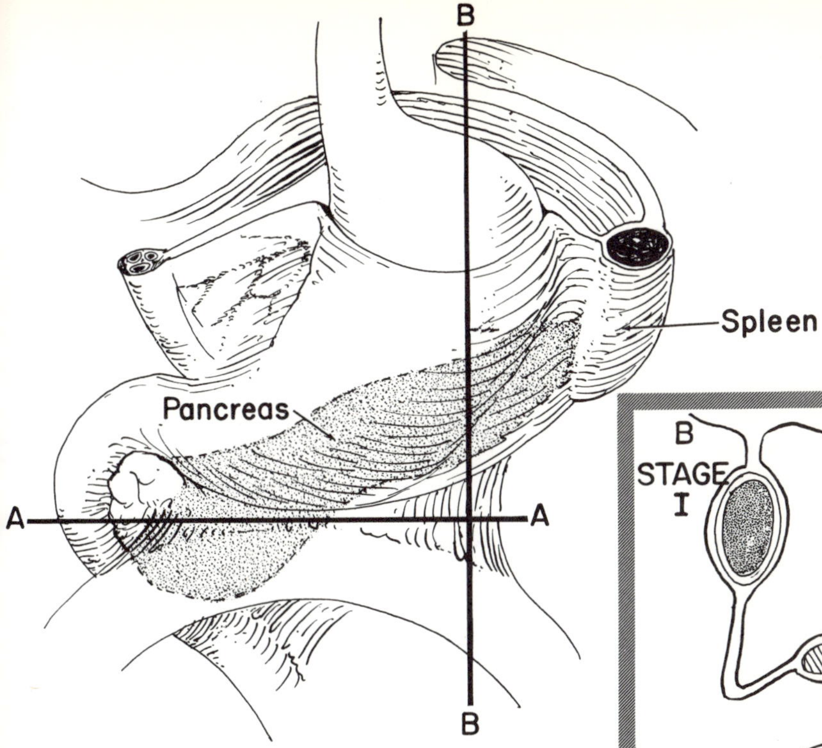

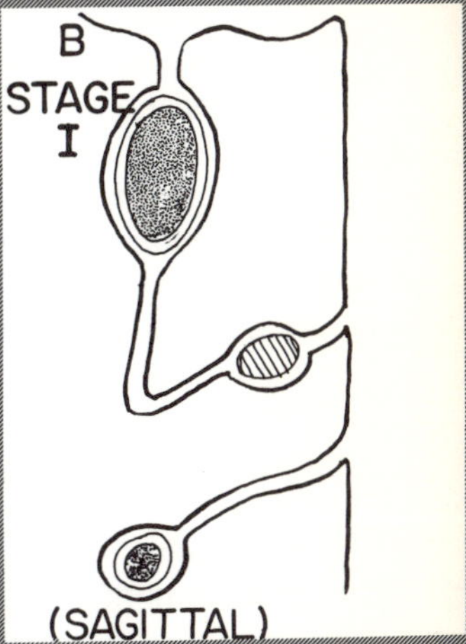

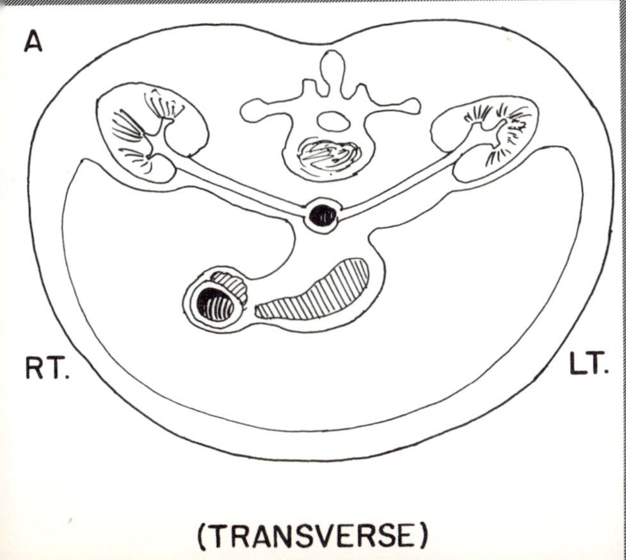

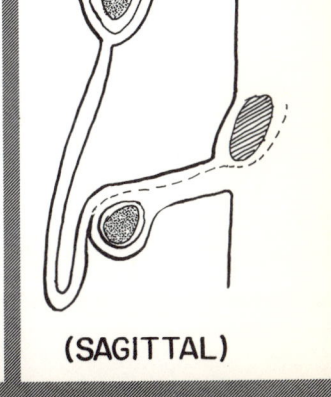

The two arterial arcades that supply the head of the pancreas are derived from the gastroduodenal and superior mesenteric arteries. They are named the anterior superior pancreaticoduodenal artery and the posterior superior pancreaticoduodenal artery. The body and tail of the pancreas are supplied by the superior pancreatic branch of the celiac artery, the inferior pancreatic branch of the superior mesenteric and several branches of the splenic and left gastroepiploic arteries **(A)**.

The venous drainage of the pancreas follows the arterial supply. The anterior and posterior pancreaticoduodenal arcades from the head of the pancreas drain into the portal and superior mesenteric veins. The veins from the body and the tail drain into the splenic, the superior and the inferior mesenteric veins. The head of the pancreas shares a common blood supply with the first and second portions of the duodenum. Similarly, the spleen shares a common blood supply with the body and the tail. It is for these reasons that resection of the tail and body is facilitated by a concomitant splenectomy and that the head of the pancreas cannot be resected entirely without a simultaneous duodenectomy.

The lymphatics of the pancreas **(B)** drain into the splenic, celiac, superior mesenteric, subpyloric and transverse mesocolic nodal basins.

The pancreas is innervated by sympathetic and parasympathetic nerves through the celiac plexus. The sympathetic supply reaches the plexus through the greater, lesser and least splanchnic nerves. The parasympathetic fibers are derived from the vagi and terminate in the intrinsic pancreatic ganglia.

Afferent pain sensation is transmitted by the sympathetic fibers through the celiac plexus to the splanchnic nerves and to the sympathetic ganglia bilaterally. The celiac ganglia lie in close proximity to and on the surface of the celiac axis, which arises from the aorta just distal to the diaphragm and the dorsal border of the body of the pancreas. Excision of the celiac plexus or its injection with alcohol may relieve pain of pancreatic origin.

The least accessible portion of the pancreas is the uncinate process, located between the superior mesenteric artery and the aorta. It is usually the last portion of the pancreas resected during a pancreaticoduodenectomy, since mobilization and excision of the duodenum facilitates its exposure. One can also gain access to it after a

PLATE 31

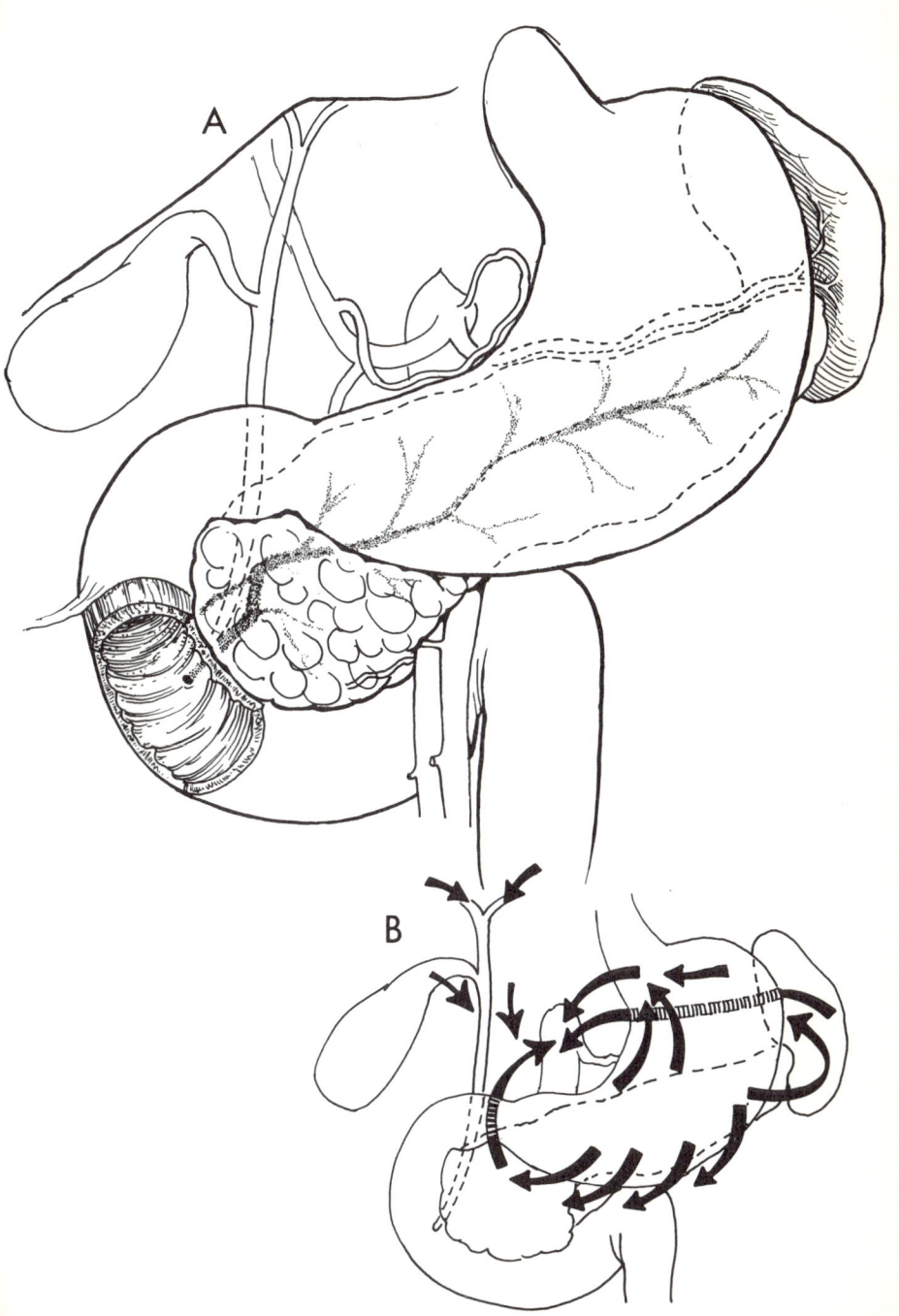

90% pancreatectomy, once the superior mesenteric vessels have been "unroofed."

Operative Approaches to the Pancreas

The incision is predicated on the physical characteristics of the patient and the preference of the surgeon.

The midline incision **(A)** is far quicker and is preferred in asthenic patients with a narrow angle between the costal margins and a thin abdominal wall. Adequate exposure is obtained by extending the incision below the umbilicus.

The transverse (inverted U) incision **(B)** is preferred in the plethoric patient with a broad chest and a thick body wall.

The choice of the particular incision is based upon a number of factors, consisting of an enumeration of the virtues and disadvantages of the longitudinal and transverse incisions. The midline incision is far quicker and creates much less dead space when the wound is closed. It is essentially a 1-layer closure. However, postoperative stress is far greater on a vertical than on a transverse incision. Transverse incisions allow for greater exposure in patients with broad chests. However, they take much longer, both during the opening and closure of the incision, and produce a greater degree of tissue necrosis and a significant dead space. Both of these factors predispose to wound infections. In rare situations, only 1 limb of the transverse incision is made; this permits exploration of the abdomen. The incision is extended as required.

[Operative approaches to the pancreas *continued on page 146.*]

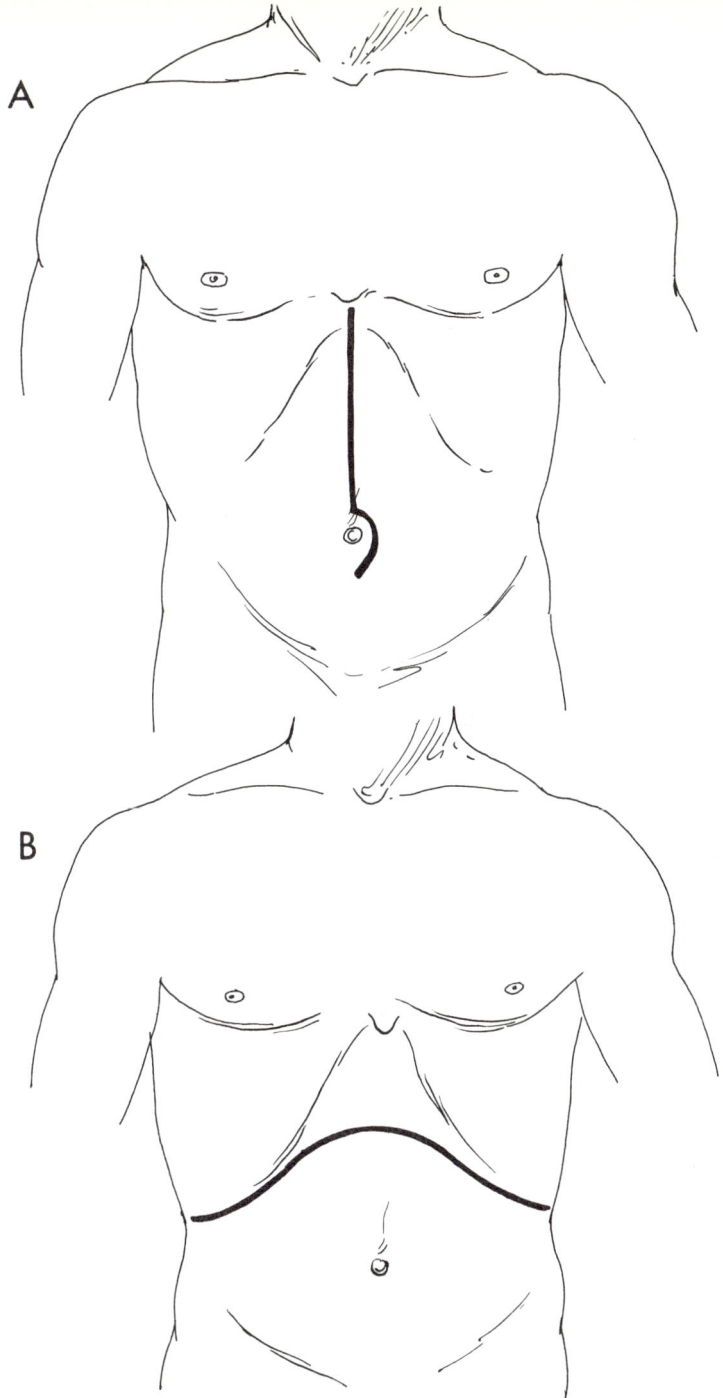

When the incision has been made and the abdomen explored, there are 3 principal avenues the surgeon can choose to expose the pancreas.

In the asthenic patient, with little or no omental fat, the lesser curvature of the stomach can be retracted in a caudad direction and the avascular portions of the gastrohepatic ligament divided. This exposes the celiac axis, the splenic artery and vein and the superior aspect of the body and tail of the pancreas **(C)**. This is the most direct approach for excisional biopsies of enlarged nodes along the superior border of the pancreas.

Exposure of the body and the tail of the pancreas is obtained by the division of the gastrocolic ligament **(D)**. This exposes the lesser peritoneal space and the entire body, the tail and a portion of the anterior surface of the head.

Another approach to the pancreas is through the transverse mesocolon **(E)**. This is done by lifting the omentum and the transverse colon, locating the middle colic and superior mesenteric vessels and opening the transverse mesocolon to the left of the middle colic vessels. This avenue provides a rapid access to subpancreatic and superior mesenteric-aortic lymph nodes. By gentle dissection of this area one can also determine the presence of a tumor in the uncinate process or head after a Kocher maneuver has been performed and the posterior surface of the head of the pancreas has been mobilized. The surgeon can then place his left hand on the posterior surface of the head of the pancreas and his right hand at the anterior surface and the inferior border of the head along the superior mesenteric vessels.

PLATE 32

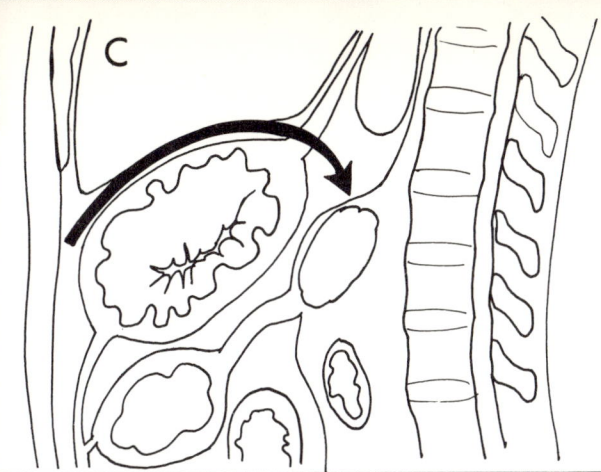

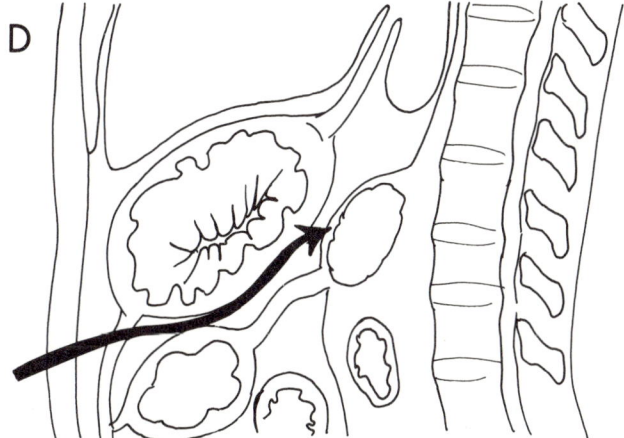

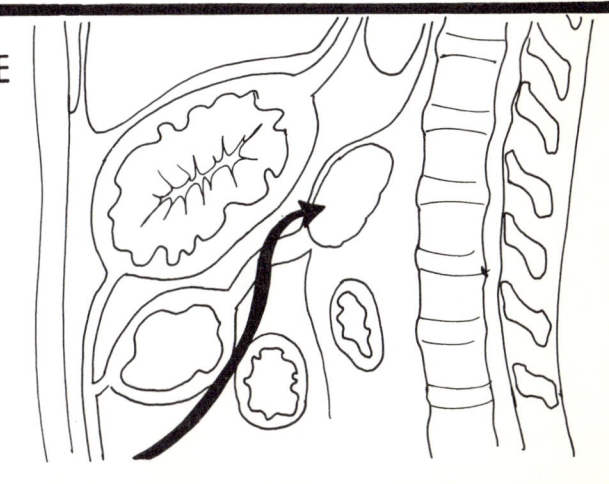

Exposure by Division of Gastrocolic Ligament

The avascular segment left to the midline is located and tented.

Through an opening at this point the surgeon places 2 fingers into the lesser peritoneal space and then divides this ligament first toward the left and then toward the right, after ligation of the intervening blood vessels **(A)**. Care is taken to preserve the gastroepiploic vessels and the integrity of the transverse colon and its blood supply. In some instances a few of the short gastric vessels must be divided to expose the entire tail of the pancreas.

Cephalad retraction is applied to the stomach by placing a Harrington retractor on its posterior surface; this exposes the splenic vessels and the celiac axis **(B)**.

The pancreas can be mobilized further by making an incision in the posterior fusion fascia at the inferior border of the body and tail. Care must be taken to preserve the inferior mesenteric vein, which courses posterior to the body of the pancreas to this point.

[Exposure of body and tail of pancreas *continued on page 150.*]

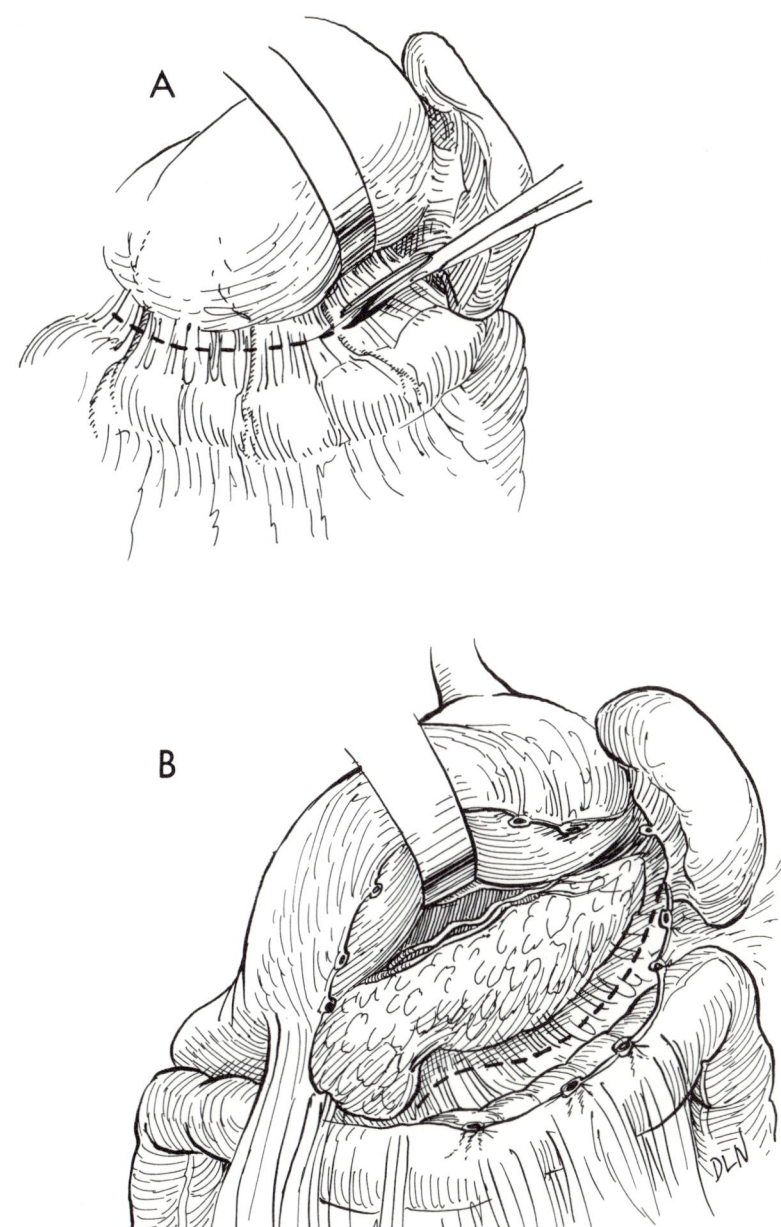

PLATE 33

Exposure of Body and Tail of Pancreas

Partial mobilization of the neck of the pancreas can be achieved by developing the potential avascular space between the neck and the anterior surface of the superior mesenteric vessels, slightly to the left **(C)**. This space will admit the index finger or a soft rubber drain for traction. Great care and gentle technic must be used in the dissection of this space, since aberrant vessels, especially in the event of previous inflammation, may exist and cause a tear in the superior mesenteric or portal vein and troublesome bleeding.

At this point, the surgeon is in an excellent position to examine the entire body and tail of the pancreas and to evaluate the celiac, dorsal pancreatic, hepatic, superior mesenteric and preaortic lymph nodes **(D)**.

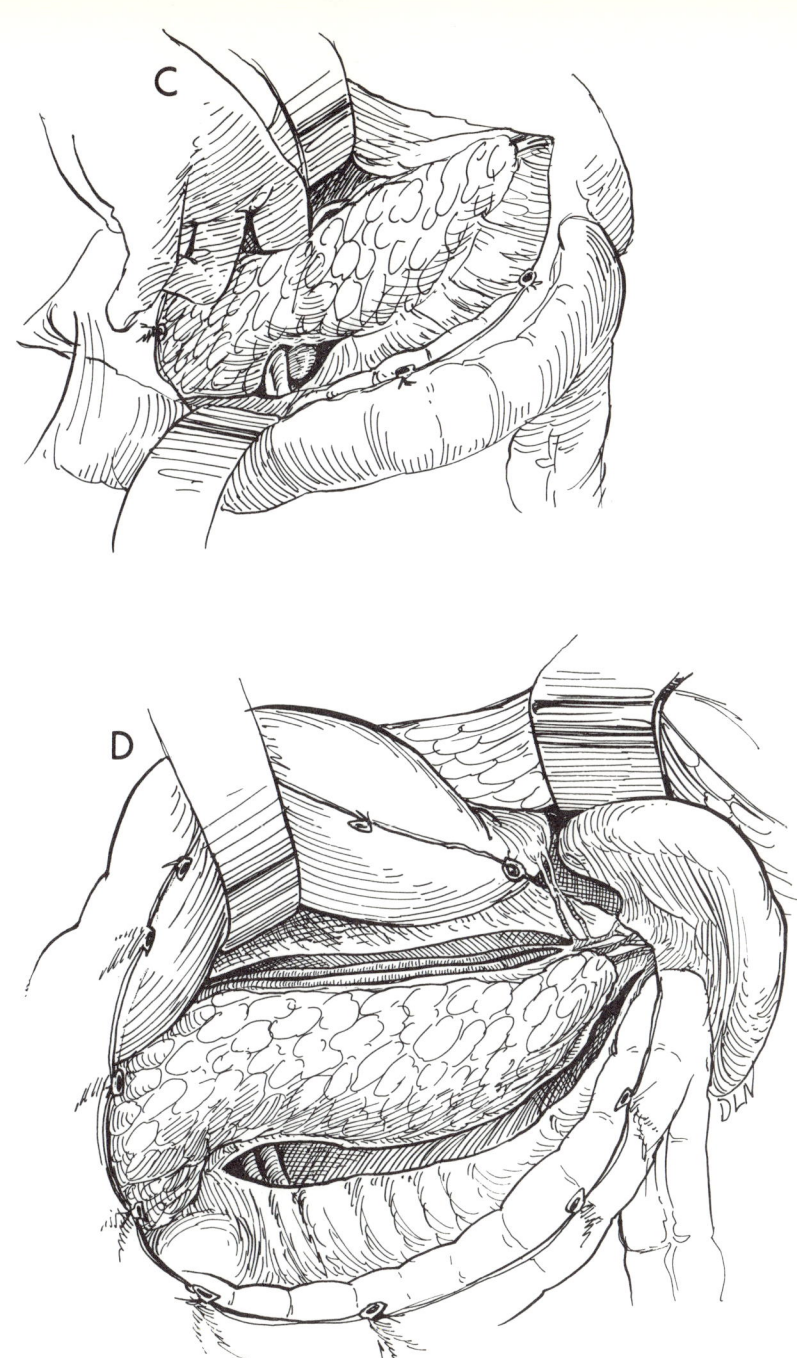

PLATE 33

Exposure and Examination of Head and Uncinate Process

Mobilization of the head of the pancreas and the first, second and third portions of the duodenum can be obtained by a simple Kocher maneuver and blunt dissection at the posterior surface of the head of the pancreas **(A)**. By this technic the head of the pancreas can be literally lifted away from the vena cava and aorta and its posterior surface to the left border of the inferior vena cava can be exposed, visualized and examined **(B)**.

Nodules within the head of the pancreas can be detected by placing the left hand on the posterior surface and the right hand along the lesser curvature of the duodenum **(C)** or in the lesser peritoneal space just to the right of the superior mesenteric vessels, or below the transverse mesocolon along and behind the partially dissected superior mesenteric vessels.

In the absence of chronic or acute inflammation, the surgeon can actually grasp the entire head of the pancreas between his thumb on the anterior surface of the head along the lesser curvature of the duodenum and his other fingers on the posterior surface of the gland **(D)**.

Nodules in the uncinate process are best detected by placing the left hand on the posterior surface of the head of the pancreas, near its inferior border, and the right hand along and behind the partially dissected superior mesenteric vessels, beneath the transverse mesocolon.

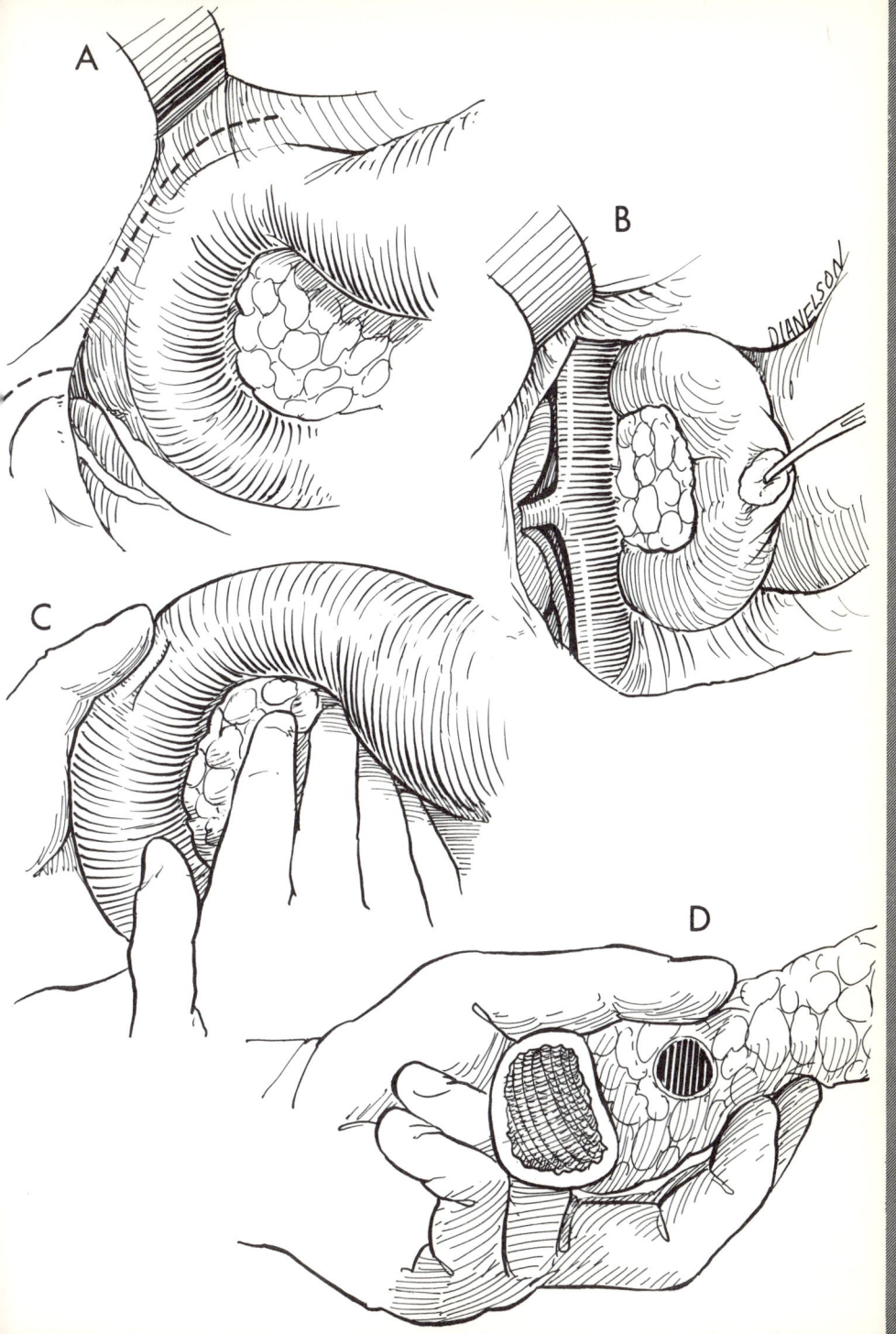

PLATE 34

Islet Cell Tumors: Biopsy

The objective of all the preceding dissections and examinations is to locate an islet cell tumor(s), which may be on the surface of the gland or within its substance and covered with normal parenchyma.

In patients with insulinomas, the objective is to find and excise the offending tumor or to do an appropriate resection if multiple tumors or adenomatous hyperplasia are found (Plate 37).

In patients with gastrinomas, the objective is to establish a tissue diagnosis of islet cell tumors and then to proceed with a total gastrectomy. This can be done in 1 of 3 ways: biopsy of a liver metastasis **(A)**, excision of a lymph node containing metastases **(B)**, and incisional or excisional biopsy of the primary tumor. Biopsy of the primary tumor is the least desirable method, since it requires manipulation and incision into the pancreas, which may set the stage for postoperative acute pancreatitis.

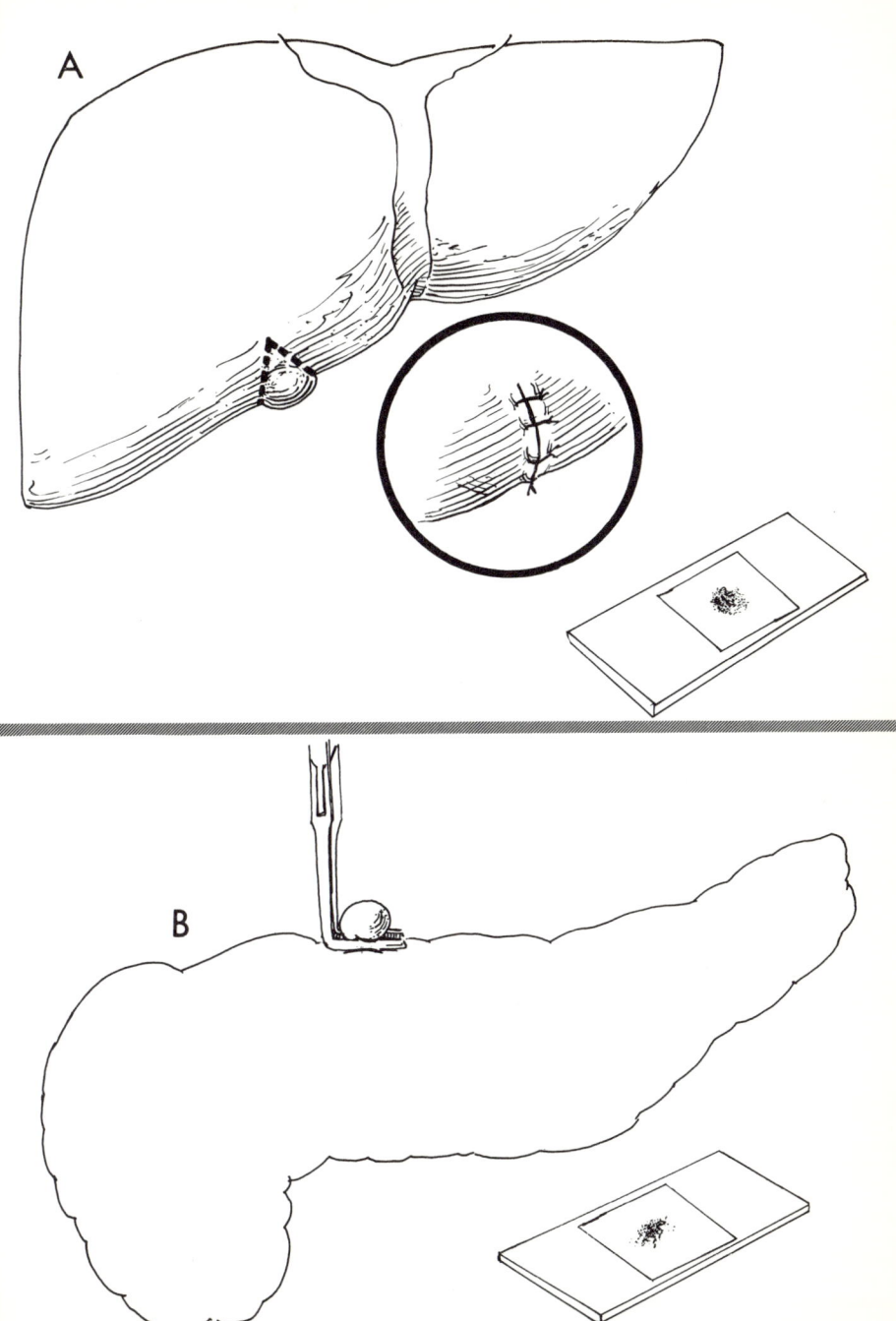

PLATE 35

Clinical Manifestations

The astute clinician will suspect the presence of hypoglycemia primarily from the history and confirmatory physical signs such as obesity in patients with functioning beta cell tumors. However, these symptoms are usually subtle and intermittent and frequently attributed to psychosomatic disturbances. There is extensive evidence indicating that the manifestations of hypoglycemia are the result of decreased cerebral metabolism, since the chief source of energy for brain tissue is glucose. The brain cannot store glucose or glycogen in significant amounts. For this reason irreversible cerebral damage is apt to occur if hypoglycemia continues beyond an interval of 1 hour. The principal symptoms and signs of hypoglycemia are:

Loss of consciousness	Drowsiness and stupor
Confused state	Lightheadedness
Weakness and fatigue	Visual disturbances
Deep coma	Amnesia
Diaphoresis	Convulsions

The symptom complex may be suggestive of:

1. Autonomic nervous system overactivity, which may be related to a compensatory release of catecholamines with accompanying fatigue, weakness, apprehension, hunger, tremor, excessive diaphoresis and tachycardia.

2. Central nervous system disturbances, such as apathy, irritability, anxiety, somnambulism, confusion, excitement, disorientation and speech, visual and behavioral defects.

Differential Diagnosis

The documentation of hypoglycemia is a relatively simple task compared to the determination of its etiology. The list of hypoglycemic syndromes is a long one; they can be classified into 4 principal categories:

1. Reactive (postabsorptive) hypoglycemia
2. Fasting hypoglycemia with deficient glucose production
3. Fasting hypoglycemia with overutilization of glucose
4. Pharmacogenic and toxic hypoglycemia

The reactive postabsorptive hypoglycemia category includes patients with latent diabetes mellitus and patients with postgastric operation syndromes.

Fasting hypoglycemia with deficient glucose production is found in patients with acquired liver disease such as alcoholic cirrhosis, patients with endocrine organ hypofunction and deficiency of glucocorticoids, glucagon or thyroid hormone secretion and patients with extrapancreatic neoplasms such as mesotheliomas and carcinomas.

Fasting hypoglycemia with overutilization of glucose is seen primarily in patients with pancreatic beta cell tumors or growth hormone deficiency and in newborn babies of diabetic mothers.

Pharmacogenic and toxic hypoglycemia is caused by the factitious or iatrogenic administration of exogenous insulin, oral hypoglycemics and ethyl alcohol.

Insulinomas

The clinical manifestations of functioning beta cell tumors are similar to the symptom complex described for hypoglycemia. These tumors are most frequent in the fourth, fifth and sixth decades, with equal sex distribution, and may have, by history, existed for years before the diagnosis is suspected and established. Although the symptoms may occur sporadically, seemingly unrelated to meals, they usually appear before breakfast and are ameliorated by food intake. In contrast, they may be precipitated by prolonged fasting or vigorous physical exercise. In some instances the decline of blood sugar may be so gradual that the release of catecholamines is blunted and, as a consequence, profound hypoglycemia occurs with loss of consciousness and depression of vasomotor function as the primary manifestations. Finally, the hunger and ensuing obesity of the classic textbook description are no longer considered distinguishing features of this syndrome.

DIAGNOSIS

The diagnosis of insulinoma depends upon a series of tests and, if possible, the radiographic demonstration of a tumor blush in the pancreas, in the following sequence:
1. Documentation of hypoglycemia
2. Documentation of inappropriate levels of circulating insulin
3. Radiographic localization
4. Excision of the tumor and histopathologic confirmation.

Hypoglycemia is documented when plasma glucose is below 50 mg/100 ml and true blood glucose is below 40 mg/100 ml.

FASTING HYPOGLYCEMIA. — After a period of 12–16 hours of fasting, 80% of patients with beta cell tumors will have significant hypoglycemia with inappropriate elevation of circulating insulin. This abnormal reciprocal relationship is unique to patients with insulin-secreting islet cell tumors. Tests may have to be repeated on several occasions before this reciprocal relationship is documented. In some instances patients may have to be subjected to prolonged fasting extending up to 3 days under close supervision in the hospital before hypoglycemia may be documented.

PROVOCATIVE TESTS. — If inappropriate circulating insulin levels are not well documented by fasting, the clinician may be able to demonstrate them by 1 of 3 provocative tests:
1. Intravenous tolbutamide
2. Intravenous glucagon
3. Oral L-leucine

These tests have certain pitfalls and may be dangerous in certain circumstances. For instance, tolbutamide should not be administered to patients with fasting plasma glucose levels below 50 mg/100 ml, and the test should be terminated with the administration of 50% glucose if the patient becomes unconscious or disoriented. Rapid glucose determination with glucose oxidase strips is useful in determining that a significant fall of glucose level has occurred and in terminating the tests by the administration of intravenous parenteral glucose.

No single provocative test will establish the diagnosis of an insulinoma. For this reason, it is best to use the glucagon and tolbutamide tolerance tests on separate days and follow these by a protracted period of fasting with measurement of plasma glucose and circulating insulin. This will provide the greatest chance of documentation of inappropriate insulin secretion. These provocative tests may still fail to document inappropriate circulating hyperinsulinism, since some insulinomas secrete insulin only episodically. For this reason, in the final analysis, the timely measurement of insulin during episodes of spontaneous fasting hypoglycemia remains the most important evidence of an insulinoma in the differential diagnosis of hypoglycemia.

DIAZOXIDE SUPPRESSION TEST. — The documentation of inappropriate insulin secretion is further substantiated by the demonstration of the depression of plasma insulin in response to the intravenous administration of diazoxide in a hypoglycemic patient. The importance of this test is that is dissipates any doubt regarding the source of the high levels of immunoreactive circulating insulin and confirms that the high levels are due to pancreatic insulin and not to nonspecific cross-reactants in the assay system. Failure of plasma insulin to fall after diazoxide administration points to an error in insulin immunoassay or to the presence of a nondiazoxide-suppressible insulinoma.

Insulinomas: Localization

RADIOGRAPHIC LOCALIZATION. — Once the laboratory diagnosis of hyperinsulinism has been made, radiographic demonstration of the site of the tumor by angiographic technics, which have succeeded in visualizing tumors measuring only 10 mm, is of utmost importance, since such small tumors may not be detectable at operation even after extensive dissection of the pancreas. The marked vascularity of these tumors has allowed their demonstration in up to 80% of patients by means of selective catheterization of the celiac and superior mesenteric arteries.

In large series, single tumors have been found to be evenly distributed throughout the pancreas **(A)**: 30% occur in the head, 34% in the body and 33% in the tail; 3% are ectopic. Approximately 10% of patients have diffuse adenomatous hyperplasia.

In most series 90% of patients harbor a single adenoma; multiple tumors or microadenomatosis **(B)** is found in the remaining 10%. Approximately 10% of these tumors are malignant and metastasize to the liver and regional lymph nodes most frequently. Capillary invasion and metastases are the prerequisites for the diagnosis of malignancy. The majority of tumors measure 10–50 mm in diameter. Ectopic sites are located along the gastrointestinal tract.

PLATE 36

A

(Ectopic 3%)

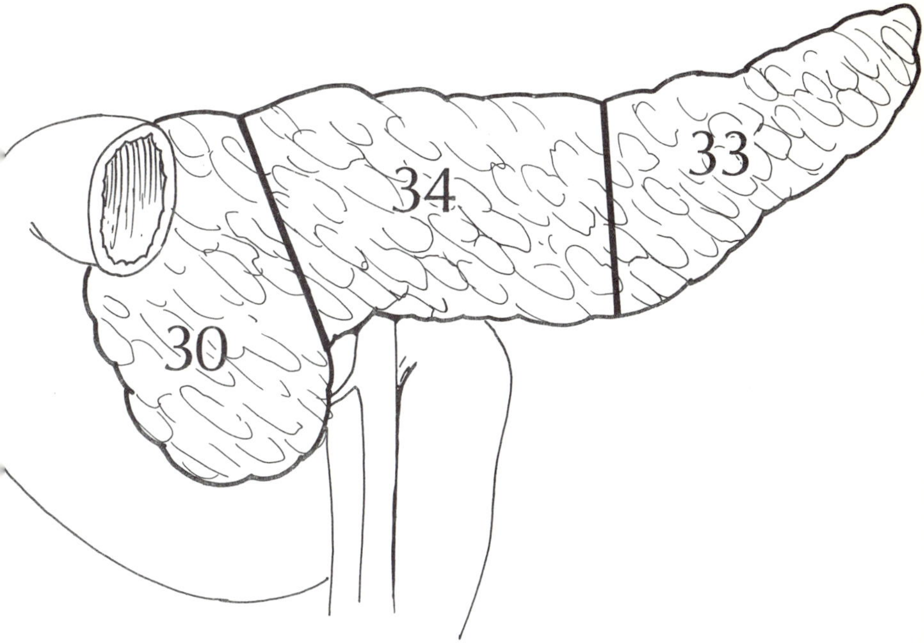

30 34 33

B

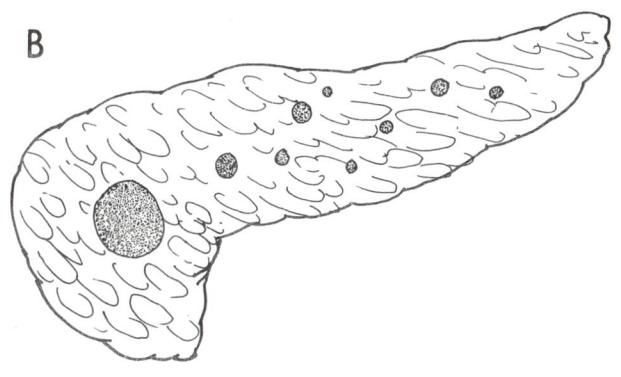

Insulinomas: Treatment

If there are no medical contraindications to a laparotomy, excision of insulinomas is the treatment of choice and usually results in a cure.

The preoperative parenteral administration of glucose, with or without glucocorticoids, has been advocated as a routine measure against hypoglycemia. The same objective can be achieved by the oral administration of diazoxide. When diazoxide is administered, the last dose should be given approximately 36 hours before operation, since the effects of this drug may persist for as long as 24 hours after the last dose. Parenteral glucose can be administered in the remaining interval. Then, whenever the return of hypoglycemia is desired, the glucose infusion can be discontinued.

Starting the operation with a rather low blood sugar will permit "blind" localization of the insulinoma when it cannot be located by palpation and visual examination of the pancreas. In such instances a stepwise resection of the pancreas, starting with the tail, accompanied by serial determinations of blood glucose, may be the only effective means of determining that the insulinoma has been resected at the moment a sharp rise of blood glucose is observed (Plate 37). Needless to say, the resected specimens are examined grossly and microscopically by frozen section during the procedure. A cross section of a fresh tissue of the pancreas may not reveal the presence of an insulinoma until the tissue is frozen, when a clear delineation of the insulinoma may occur.

This method is preferable to the 80% "blind" distal resection of the body and tail, an operation that has long been advocated as a solution to a problem that has plagued surgeons for many years. This was based on the assumption that most insulinomas were located in the body or the tail. Actually, occult tumors, which evade detection, are more likely to be in the head or uncinate process, since those are the portions where the pancreas is thickest and most difficult to examine and palpate.

PLATE 37

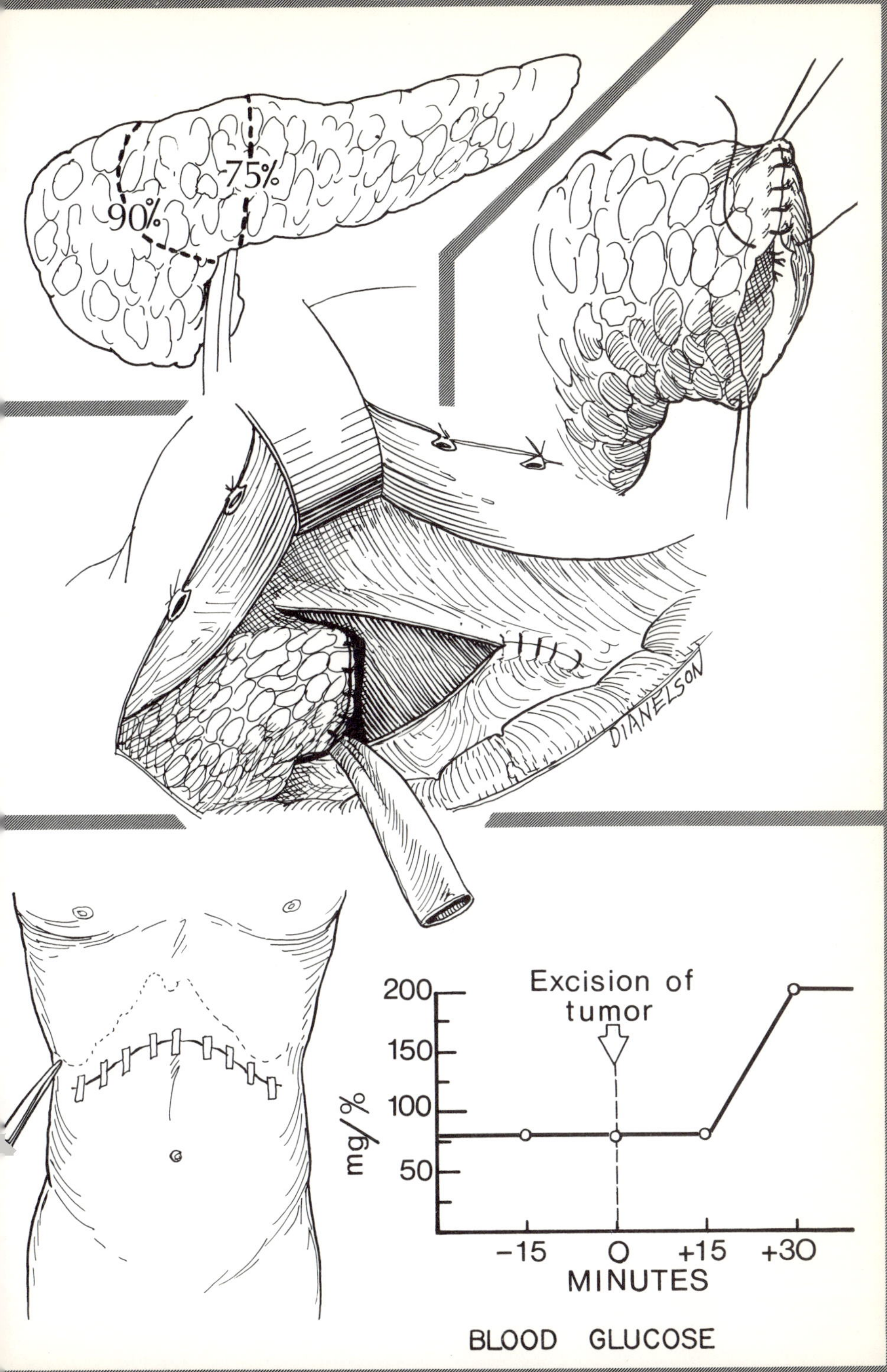

90%   75%

Excision of tumor

200
150
100
50

mg/%

−15   0   +15   +30
MINUTES

BLOOD GLUCOSE

Tumors in Body or Tail of Pancreas

Once the tumor is located within the body or the tail of the pancreas through an opening into the gastrocolic ligament, the entire length of the body and the tail of the pancreas is exposed by division of this ligament from the splenic hilus on the left to the superior mesenteric vessels on the right **(A)**.

The infrapancreatic fusion fascia is divided. Care is taken to avoid injury to the inferior mesenteric vein, which crosses posterior to the pancreas in this region.

The site of pancreatic transection is selected. This is usually just to the left of the superior mesenteric vessels **(B)**.

By very gentle and careful blunt dissection, the usually avascular space between the anterior surface of the superior mesenteric vessels and the posterior surface of the body of the pancreas is developed **(C)**. A Penrose drain may be passed through this space, around the body of the pancreas, to apply gentle traction and to facilitate further dissection.

[Resection for tumors in body or tail of pancreas *continued on page 166.*]

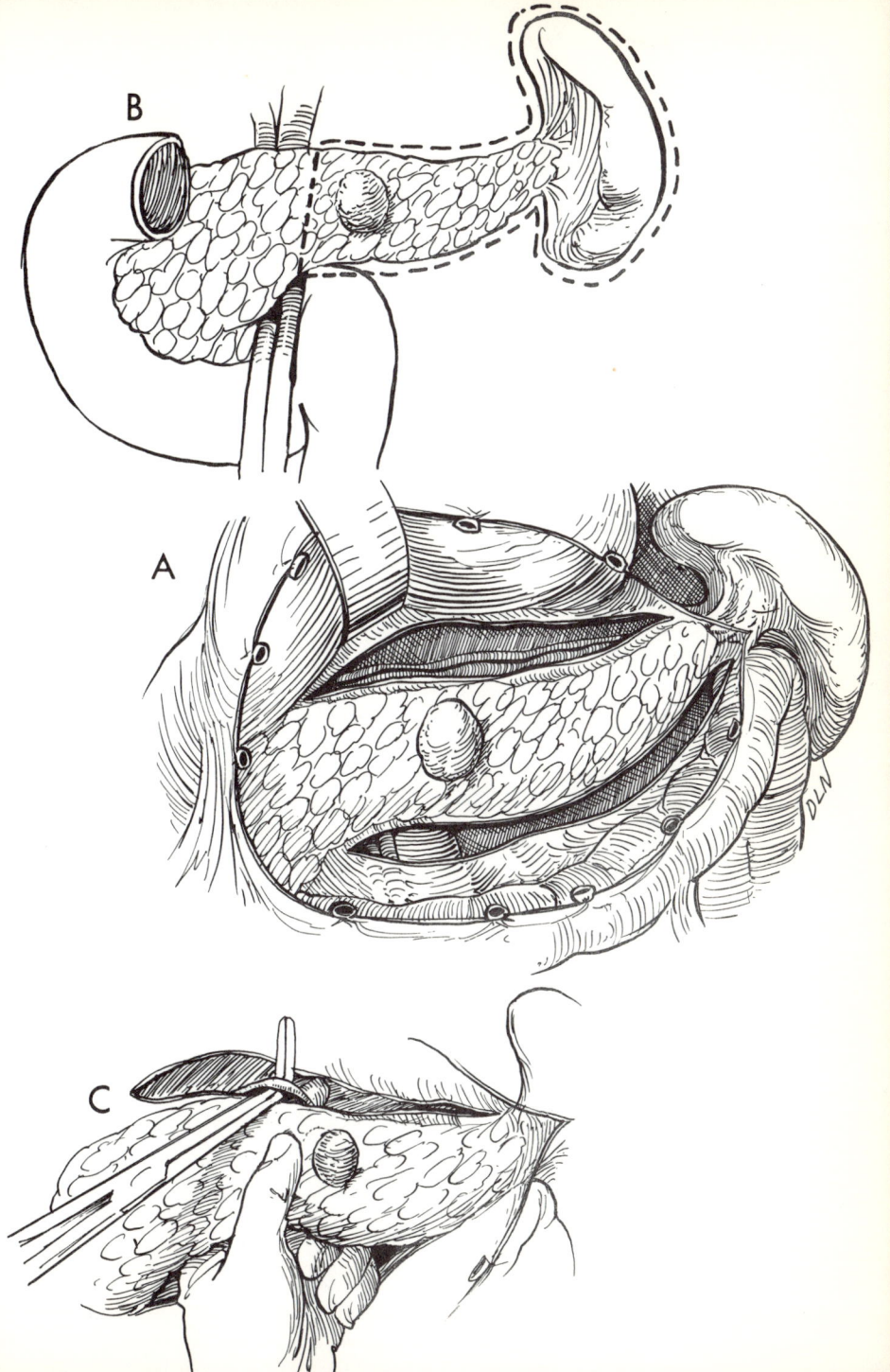

The next step is to dissect the splenic vein and artery and to divide them between double ligatures **(D)**. This procedure will minimize the degree of inadvertent bleeding that may occur during the remainder of the dissection, which includes the spleen and the tail of the pancreas.

Attention now is turned to the spleen, which is reflected medially **(E)**. The lienophrenic, lienocolic and splenorenal ligaments are exposed and individually divided. These ligaments are generally avascular; however, vessels, especially veins of substantial size, may course through them, particularly after pre-existing inflammatory processes. Painstaking hemostasis is of the utmost importance to minimize the chances of postoperative complications such as abscesses and pancreatitis.

[Resection for tumors in body or tail of pancreas *continued on page 168.*]

PLATE 38

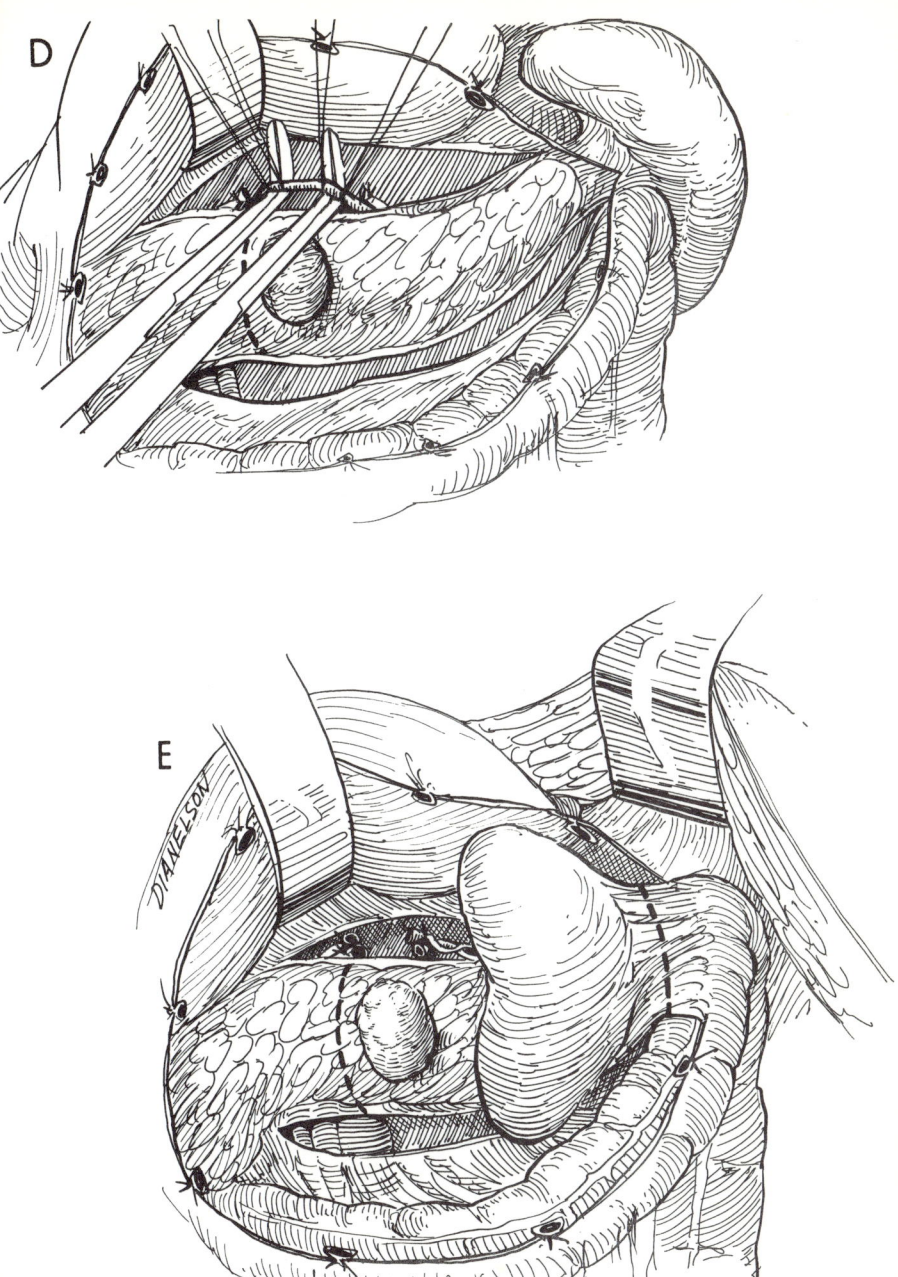

Tumors in Body or Tail of Pancreas

The surgeon turns his attention to the short gastric vessels, which are divided between ligatures, very close to the splenic hilus **(F)**.

The spleen and the tail of the pancreas are now ready to be lifted and retracted medially. The dissection proceeds along the posterior surface of the pancreas, which can now be well visualized. This is usually an avascular plane. Great care is exerted to avoid injury to the inferior mesenteric vessels, the left adrenal gland and its vein. Once the entire circumference of the pancreas has been dissected at the point which had been preselected for transection, stay sutures are placed on the capsule, superiorly and inferiorly **(G)**. The gland is transected stepwise; bleeding points are individually suture-ligated with nonabsorbable material. The central duct and its accompanying artery are individually ligated **(H)**.

[Closure *on page 170.*]

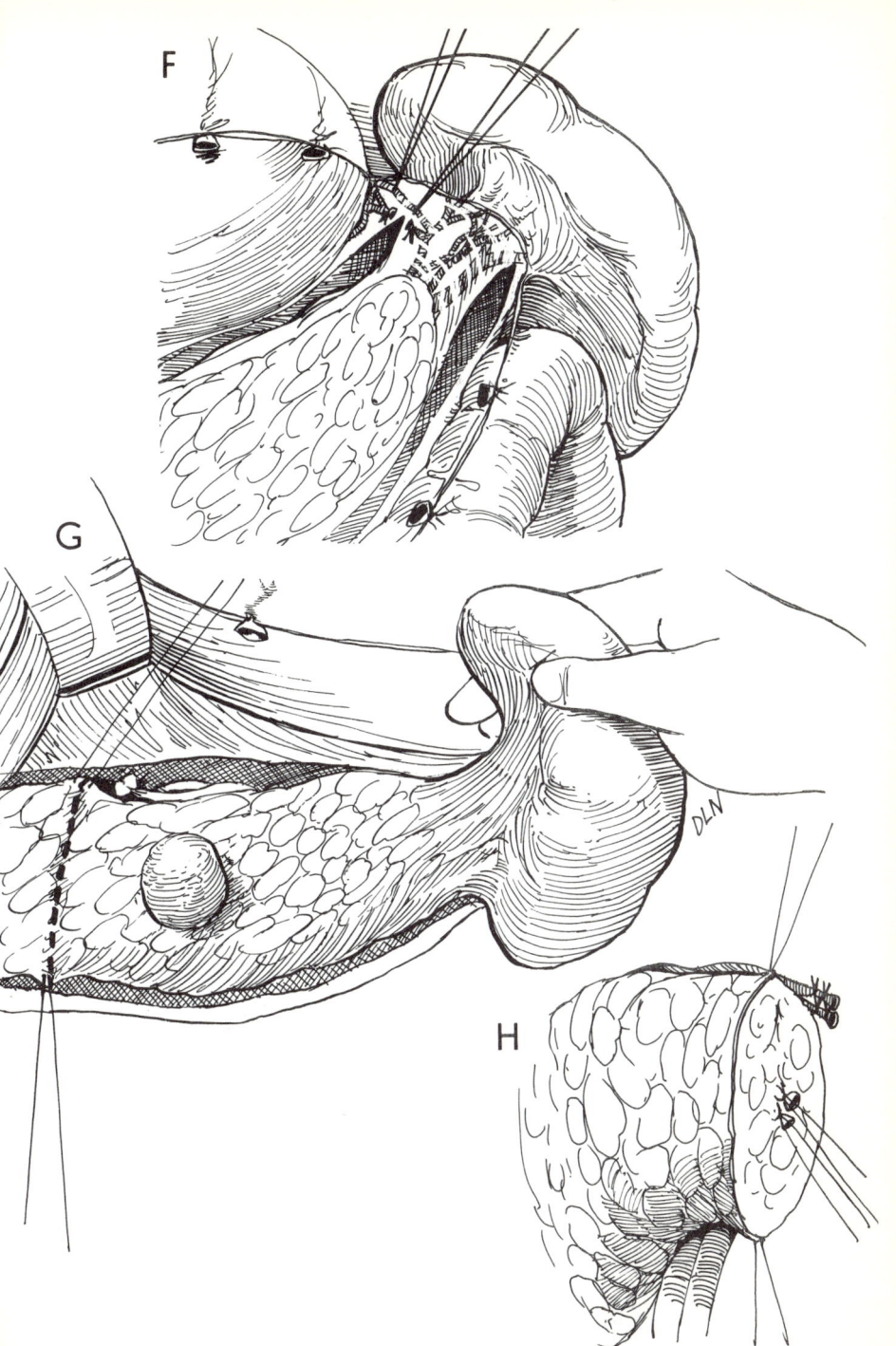

The cross-sectional defect of the pancreas is closed by approximating the anterior and posterior surface capsules with interrupted nonabsorbable sutures **(I)**. This can be done in 1 or 2 layers. In some situations it is technically impossible to infold substantial amounts of parenchyma without creating extensive necrosis of pancreatic tissue and setting the stage for postoperative acute pancreatitis. Significant leakage of pancreatic juice from the small duct radicles will occur only if there is proximal obstruction to the flow of pancreatic juice into the duodenum. Nevertheless, adequate extraperitoneal drainage is utilized. A large, soft rubber drain **(J)** is left in situ for at least 10 days to create a channel surrounded by collagen tissue, which will persist after the drain is removed **(K)**. In the event of late postoperative collections of fluid or abscess formation, which might elude recognition and diagnosis, this channel will provide an avenue for spontaneous drainage.

PLATE 38

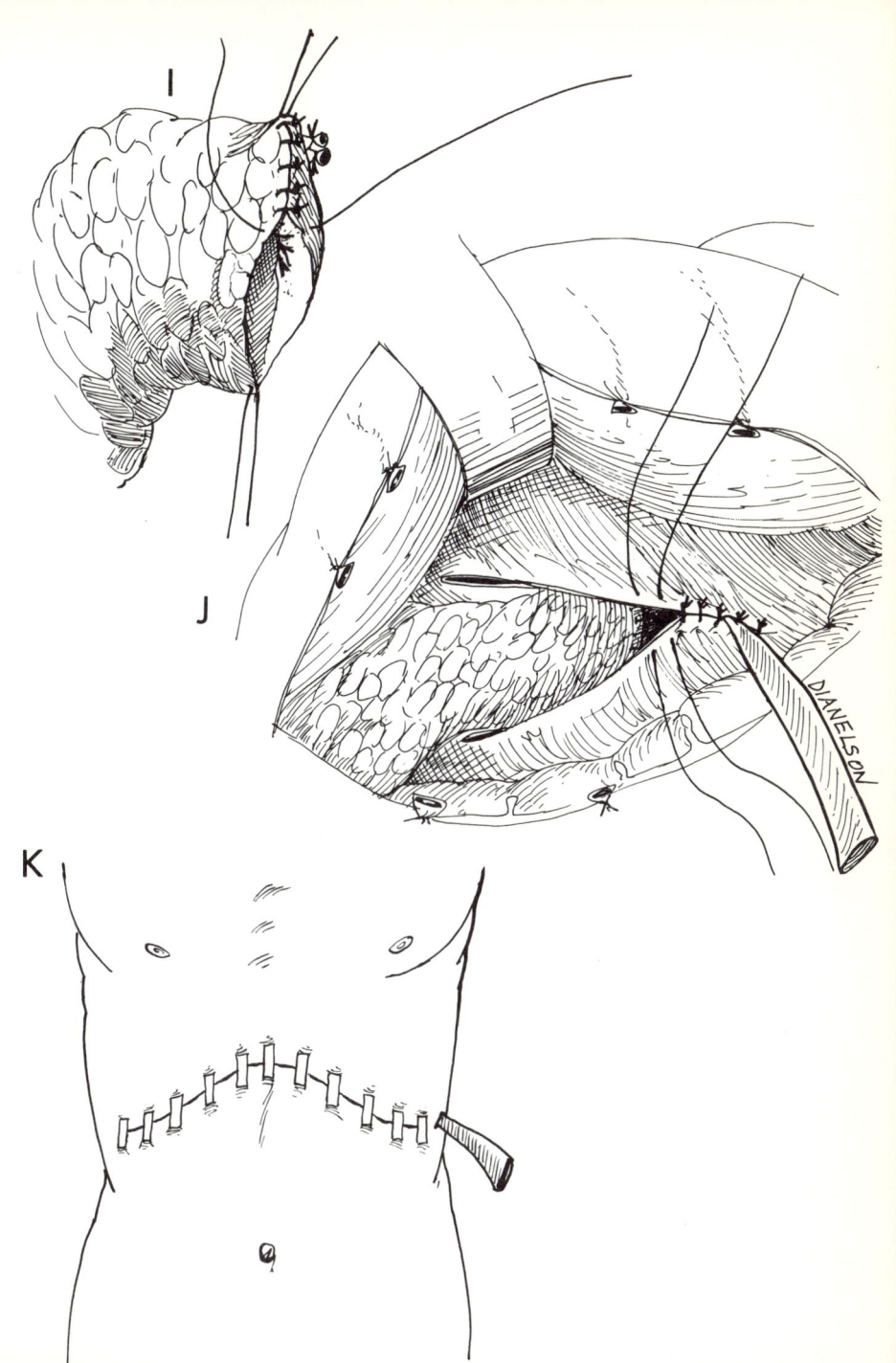

Tumors in Head of Pancreas

Enucleation is the procedure of choice for tumors located in the head of the pancreas **(A)**. Complete enucleation with minimal necrosis of pancreatic parenchyma and without damage to the main duct (and consequent obstruction of the flow of pancreatic juice) is the goal. This goal can usually be achieved, since most of these tumors are 2 cm in diameter or less and are usually well delineated grossly because of their vascularity and tan-brown color, characteristic of endocrine tumors.

To evaluate the depth of the tumor and facilitate dissection, a Kocher maneuver is done **(B)**. The surgeon grasps the head of the pancreas and duodenum to stabilize these structures during the enucleation **(C)**.

[Enucleation of tumors in head of pancreas *continued on page 174.*]

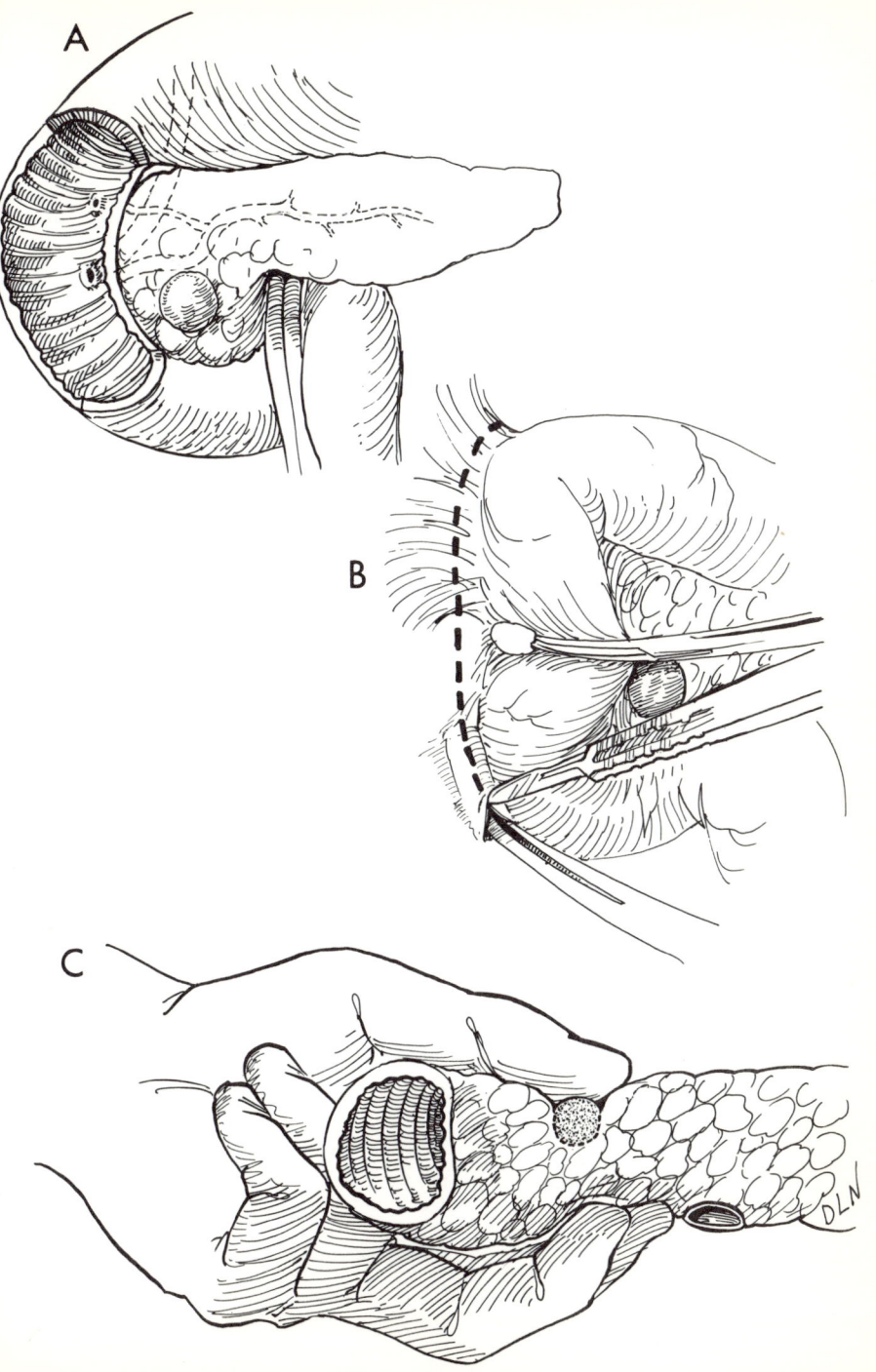

Tumors in Head of Pancreas

The surgeon places the left hand behind the head of the pancreas and the thumb on the anterior surface of the head of the pancreas and the duodenum **(D)**. With blunt and sharp dissection, and painstaking hemostasis with suture-ligatures, the tumor is gently enucleated. The surface of the pancreas is closed with interrupted nonabsorbable sutures, and extraperitoneal drainage is instituted **(E)**.

In this procedure there is no absolute method to ascertain the integrity of the duct system prior to closure. With good hemostasis and gentle dissection of the tumor, the surgeon will be able to visualize the structures he dissects and should be in a position to identify a major duct and avoid injury to it.

[Enucleation of tumors on posterior surface *on page 176.*]

PLATE 39

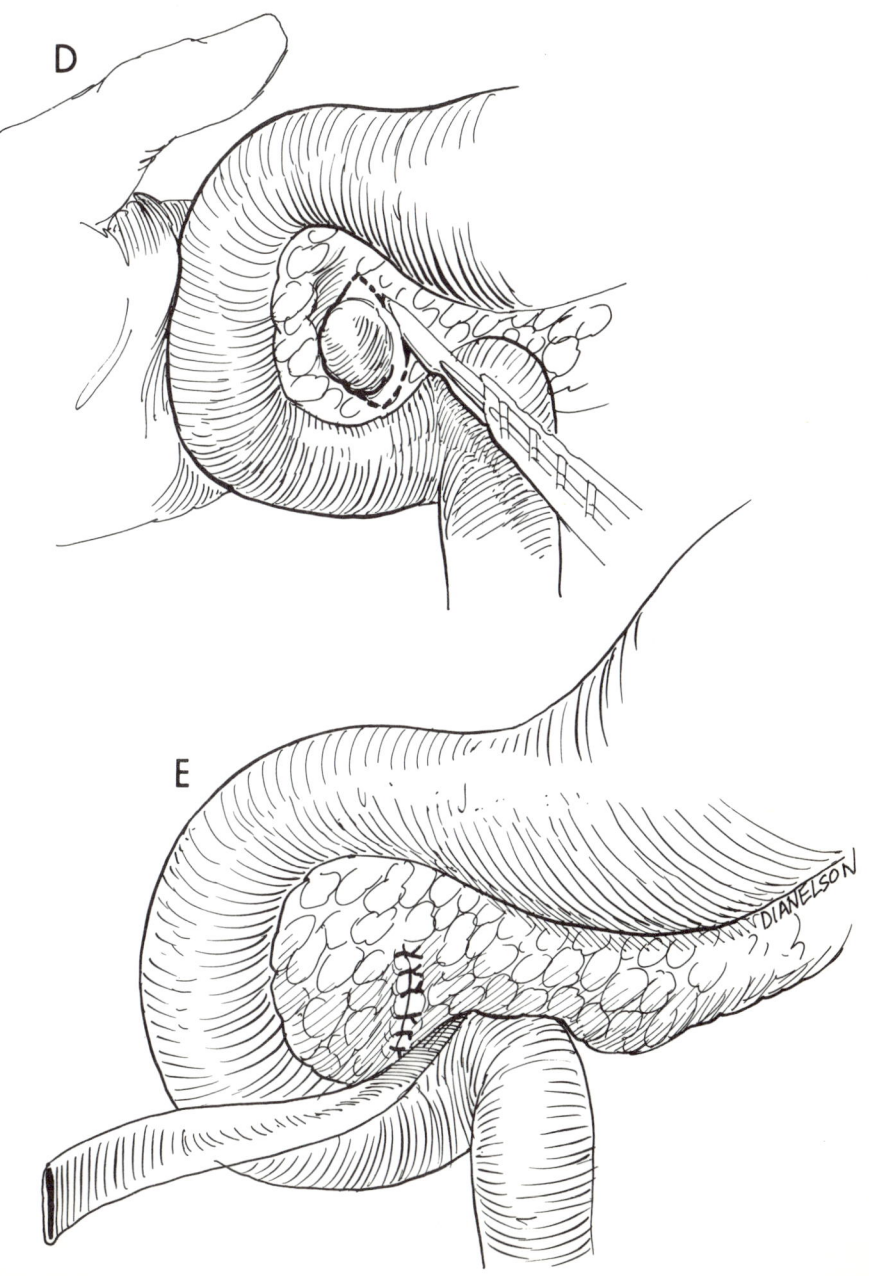

Tumors on or near the posterior surface of the head of the pancreas are also excised by enucleation with the same precautions and essentially the same technic described for tumors on the anterior surface (F–I).

Tumors within the Uncinate Process

It is almost impossible to localize tumors of the uncinate process by angiography, since they are sandwiched between the aorta posteriorly and the superior mesenteric vessels and their major branches anteriorly.

The excision of such a tumor without injury to the duodenum and bleeding from the adjacent major vessels, which include the left renal vein, the superior mesenteric vessels, the aorta, the vena cava and the pancreaticoduodenal vessels, is a technical challenge to the surgeon. Because of the difficult access to the uncinate process, it is usually the last portion of the surgical specimen excised in the course of a pancreaticoduodenectomy.

If the patient has had a previous unsuccessful pancreaticoduodenectomy with mobilization and unroofing of the superior mesenteric vessels, throwing them to the left of the aorta with bowing in an anterior direction, oblique angiographic views of the space between the aorta and superior mesenteric artery may disclose the presence of an islet cell tumor that had escaped detection in previous studies.

Access to the uncinate process is facilitated by an 80% pancreatectomy. This allows access to this area from an anterior approach. The surgeon retracts the superior mesenteric vessels toward the left and, after placing stay sutures on the pancreatic remnant, is able to expose major portions of the uncinate process by traction on the stay sutures.

With this exposure and traction, excision of the uncinate process, with adequate hemostasis, is feasible.

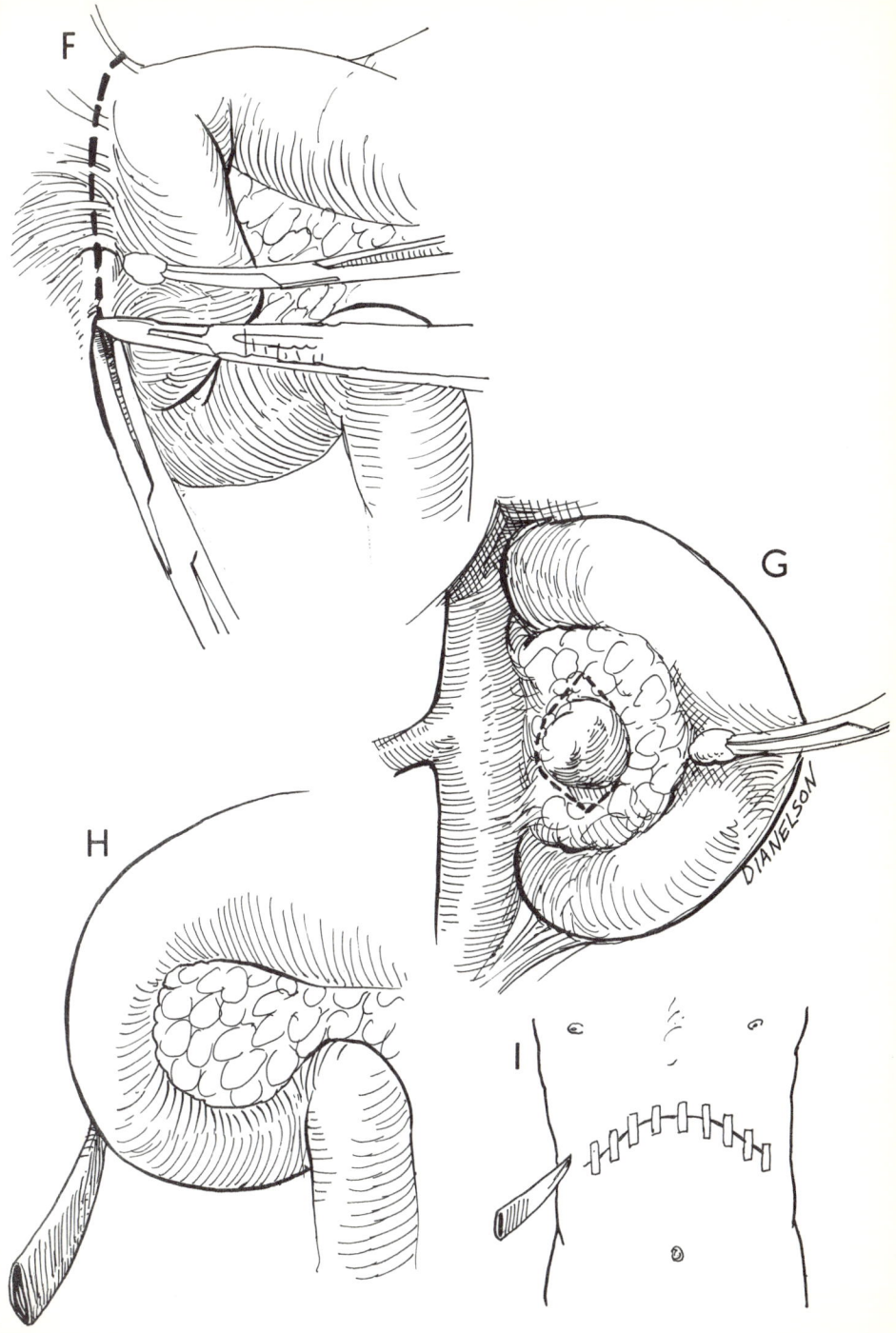

In the instance of an intraduodenal ectopic tumor **(A)**, which may have been suspected by a combination of angiography and upper gastrointestinal barium examination and actually visualized by endoscopy, the operative procedure begins with the mobilization of the duodenum and the head of the pancreas by a Kocher maneuver. This allows the surgeon to stabilize the duodenum and head of the pancreas by placing his left hand behind the duodenum. The tumor is localized by palpation if possible.

The incision line is demarcated with stay sutures, which are also used for traction. A longitudinal incision is made over the presumed location of the tumor **(B)**. Stay sutures are now placed on the 2 edges of the incision, which are retracted to expose the tumor **(C)**.

[Enucleation of ectopic tumor *continued on page 180.*]

PLATE 40

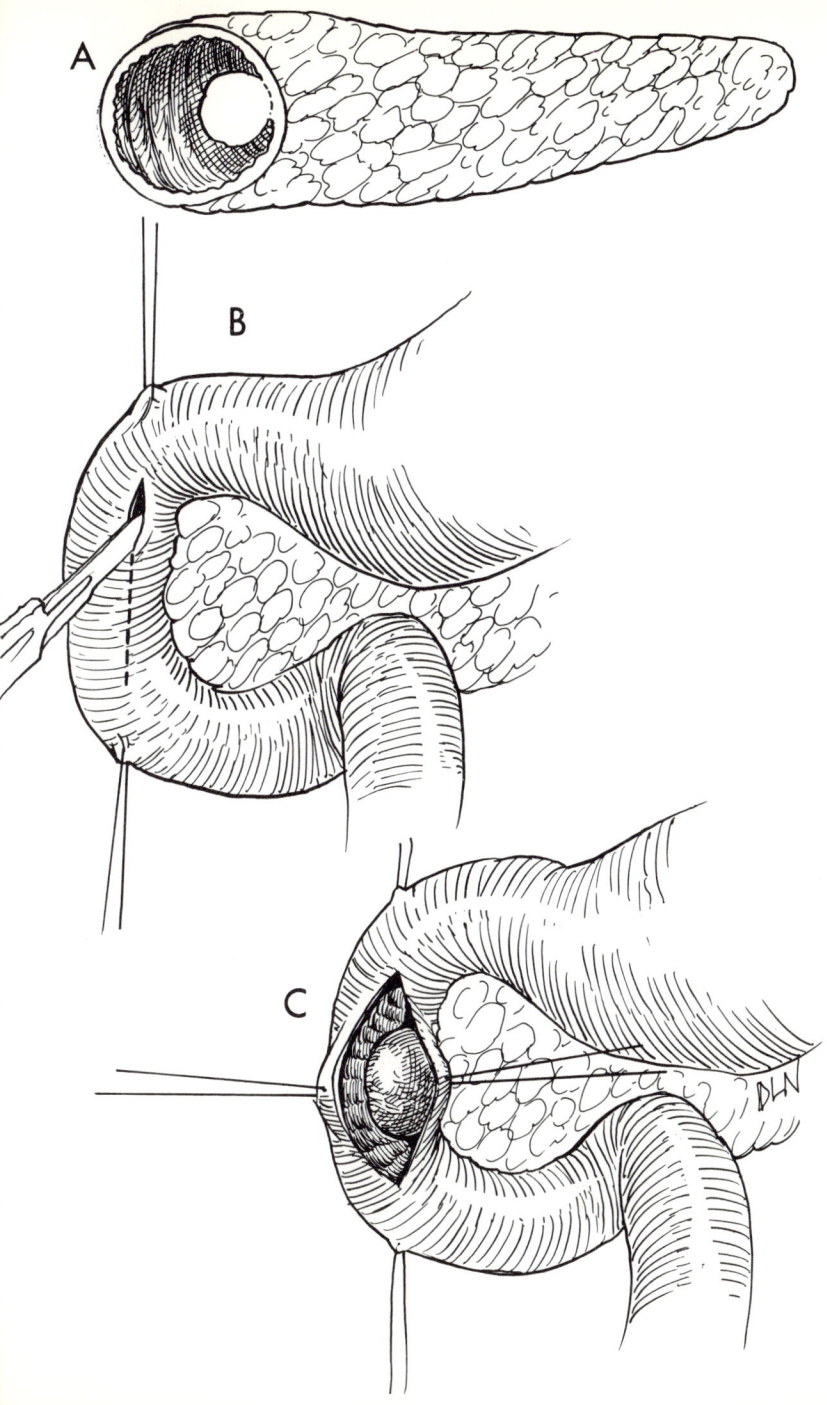

Stay sutures are placed on the duodenal mucosa at the proximal and distal end of the tumor. An elliptical incision is made in the duodenal mucosa **(D)** after the papilla of Vater has been identified and the openings of both the ducts of Wirsung and Santorini (if possible) have been located. Great care must be exercised to avoid injury or obstruction of the main duct (Wirsung) during the incision of the duodenal mucosa, the dissection and enucleation of the tumor and especially the closure of the mucosal defect **(E)**.

The surest method of ascertaining patency of the duct is to observe the brisk flow of clear pancreatic juice from the papilla **(F)** immediately after the administration of 100 units of secretin intravenously.

[Closure *on page 182.*]

PLATE 40

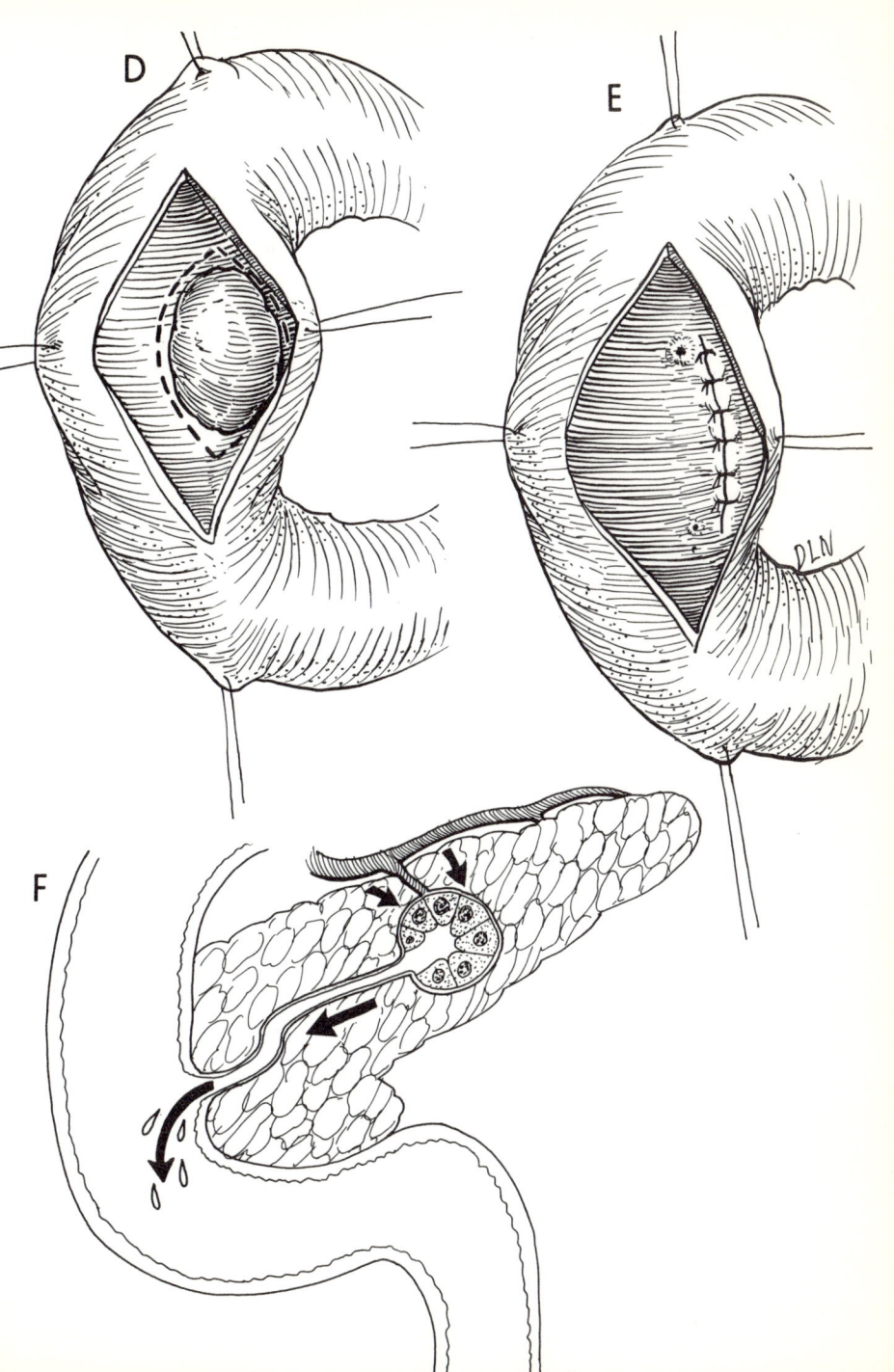

The free flow of pancreatic juice having been observed, the proximal and distal duodenal lumina are examined to ascertain the absence of obstruction and constriction.

The stay sutures previously placed on each side of the longitudinal incision to obtain exposure of the lumen are now utilized to place *transverse* traction on the incision. The longitudinal incision is closed transversely to avoid constriction of the lumen and the possibility of obstruction **(G)**. The incision is closed in 2 layers: an inner row of continuous inverting (Connell) stitch with 000 chromic catgut and an outer row of interrupted stitches with 0000 nonabsorbable sutures.

The duodenum at the site of the closed incision is palpated to assure patency of the lumen. The nasogastric tube within the gastric antrum is positioned once more to ascertain effective drainage of gastric and duodenal contents. The incision is closed in layers. There is no need for peritoneal drainage **(H)**.

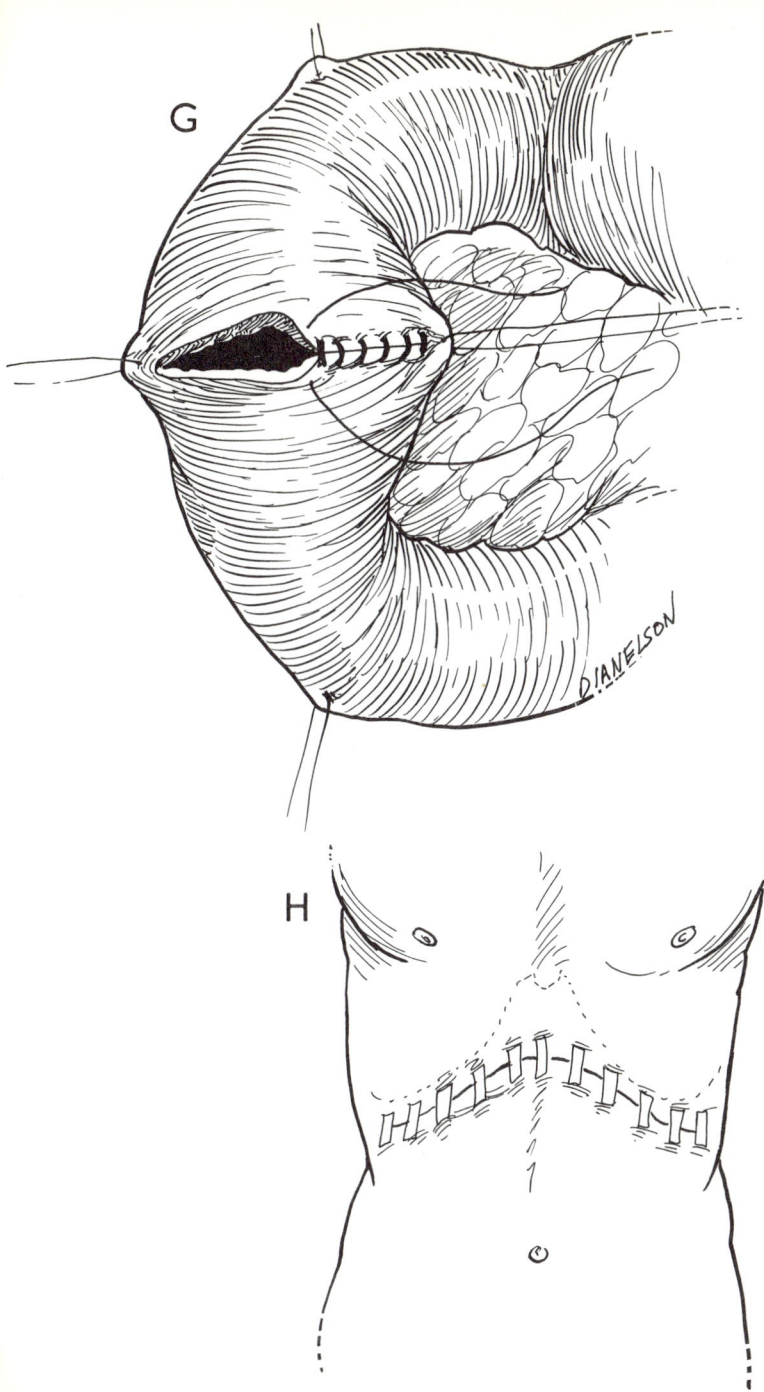

Postoperative Management of Insulinomas

Postoperative hyperglycemia, which may last 10-20 days, is a desirable result. These patients may require exogenous insulin on rare occasions.

A short-lived state of adrenal insufficiency, possibly secondary to pituitary failure, has been noted in these patients during the postoperative recovery period. The characteristic symptoms of hypotension, nausea and high fever are dramatically reversed by the administration of adrenal glucocorticoids.

In cases where hypoglycemia persists or recurs after operation, reoperation is not undertaken until the patient has recovered fully. The hypoglycemia is controlled by the administration of diazoxide. The diagnosis of hyperinsulinism is confirmed by repetition of appropriate tests. Angiographic visualization of the tumor is likely to be more successful, since a major portion of the pancreas has been resected and the radiologist can concentrate his efforts on the head and the uncinate process.

Finally, a word about operative complications. In addition to adrenal-pituitary insufficiency, acute pancreatitis is apt to develop. In large composite series, the mortality rate is reported to be 6% for first operations and 18% for second interventions.

With adequate resection, the long-term cure rate exceeds 80%.

Medical Treatment of Beta Cell Tumors

In situations in which operation may be delayed, refused or contraindicated, or in patients with metastatic insulinomas, pharmacologic control of hyperinsulinism has been available in recent years, if dietary management with frequent intake of carbohydrates fails to control the symptoms.

A number of hormones, such as long-acting zinc glucagon, glucocorticoids and epinephrine, have been tried singly or in combination; these are temporarily palliative but of little value on a long-term basis.

Diazoxide.—Effective long-term control in reliable patients has been obtained in recent years with diazoxide, a nondiuretic benzothiadiazine, which is thought to inhibit insulin release from beta cells and to enhance the secretion of epinephrine, which in turn impedes insulin secretion. Effective oral doses of diazoxide range from 300 to 750 mg daily. Side effects include gastrointestinal irritation, fluid retention and agranulocytosis. Diazoxide may be ineffective in some patients with benign insulinomas or beta cell carcinomas and in hypoglycemia due to extrapancreatic neoplasms.

Streptozotocin and metastatic tumors. — In metastatic beta cell carcinomas, alloxan, 5-fluorouracil and other chemotherapeutic agents have been ineffective.

Recently streptozotocin, an antibiotic, has been shown to be toxic to beta cells. Remission of symptomatic hypoglycemia and objective evidence of tumor regression have been demonstrated with 1 gm/m^2 body surface area, administered once a week intravenously. Side effects include nausea, vomiting, transient hepatitis and renal tubular toxicity.

EXTRAPANCREATIC NEOPLASMS

A large intrathoracic or intra-abdominal mass in the subdiaphragmatic retroperitoneal area, in conjunction with hypoglycemia and low circulating insulin levels that do not respond to insulinotropic stimuli such as tolbutamide, distinguish patients with nonpancreatic neoplasms from those with beta cell tumors. The symptoms and clinical manifestations of these patients may be remarkably similar to those of patients with beta cell tumors, however. The low circulating insulin level is the key to the differentiation, in addition to the massive proportions these tumors may reach (2–4 kg).

The pathogenesis of the hypoglycemia of these patients is speculative. Increased utilization of glucose by these large tumors and decreased glucose production secondary to substance(s) produced by these neoplasms, which inhibit hepatic gluconeogenesis and cause defective glycogen synthesis and degradation, have been advanced as possible mechanisms with fragmentary evidence.

Ordinarily these are mesenchymal tumors, classified most commonly as low-grade fibrosarcomas, fibromas, rhabdomyosarcomas and leiomyosarcomas. Their size and anatomic location usually preclude complete excision. Therapy is directed toward the maintenance of tolerable blood glucose levels, with frequent intake of carbohydrates and the administration of pharmacologic doses of glucocorticoids. Except for a few instances in which diazoxide has been of some benefit, chemotherapeutic agents and radiation therapy have been ineffective.

Gastrinomas

History

In 1955 Zollinger and Ellison described 2 patients in whom they observed the triad of (1) jejunal (ectopic) or recurrent peptic ulcer; (2) marked gastric acid hypersecretion, and (3) non-beta islet cell tumors, usually located in the pancreas. This syndrome is caused by gastrin-secreting islet cell tumors, which have been designated gastrinomas.

The clinical characterization of the Zollinger-Ellison syndrome remained confused for some years after it was first described. For example, the watery diarrhea that many of these patients exhibit was thought to be primarily due to the inactivation of gastrointestinal enzymes by the copious amounts of acid gastric juice that poured into the small bowel. In 1968 data were presented by Zollinger and co-workers that implicated a secretin-like hormone as the agent responsible for the watery diarrhea, hypokalemia and achlorhydria of the diarrheogenic syndrome. To date some 65 documented cases of this syndrome have been reported in the world literature.

Clinical Manifestations

The clinical manifestations of gastrinomas consist of severe peptic ulcer diathesis of the upper gastrointestinal tract, with marked elevations of gastric acid secretion and, in many instances, watery diarrhea. These symptoms are refractory to conventional therapeutic measures. Basal serum gastrin levels are markedly elevated.

This syndrome is most often recognized between the third and fifth decades of life. Males outnumber females by a ratio of 3:2. Untreated patients seldom survive much beyond the fifth decade. Pain occurs in 9 out of 10 patients, and usually but not always is a classic ulcer pain. There is a high rate of complications of ulcer disease, particularly hemorrhage and perforation, which occur in half the cases. With the watery diarrhea, fluid loss is notable.

Gastrinomas are an excellent example of endocrine tumors that secrete a hormone with a normal physiologic function in excess quantities, and that are controlled by directing the treatment at the target organ rather than the tumor itself. After several years of complications and failures, experience has shown that removal of the entire stomach (the target organ), which at first glance seems to be a harsh prescription, is an effective therapeutic measure, compatible with long-term survival of these patients and with minimal incapacitation. The reasons for the failure of resection of the tumor are apparent from the pathologic data: 60% of these tumors are malignant, and 70% of the malignant tumors have demonstrable metastases. Even though 40% of these tumors are benign, most of them are multiple or hyperplastic.

From the foregoing, it is obvious that even pancreaticoduodenectomy offers only a minimal chance of cure to these patients. Further, a total gastrectomy is a simple procedure and less incapacitating than pancreaticoduodenectomy.

Another fascinating facet of these gastrinomas is the report by Friesen of a small series of patients whose metastatic islet cell neoplasms have shown regression after total gastrectomy, i.e., removal of the target organ. Gastrin levels seem to decrease after total gastrectomy, even though the tumor has not been removed. This implies the possibility of a feedback mechanism governing tumor activity.

Finally, regarding the watery diarrhea in patients with gastrinomas, it now seems clear that there are at least 2 groups of patients with islet cell syndromes and watery diarrhea: (1) patients with marked gastric hypersecretion; (2) patients with achlorhydria (or hypochlorhydria) and hypokalemia caused by excess production of a nonidentified polypeptide hormone.

The differentiation is made by the finding of marked gastric acid hypersecretion in gastrinomas and the abolishment of the diarrhea by gastric aspirations and gastrectomy.

Diagnosis

The diagnosis begins with a high index of suspicion on the part of the clinician in patients who have severe peptic ulcer diathesis of the upper gastrointestinal tract or whose ulcer diathesis is refractory to the standard therapeutic measures that may have controlled their symptoms for many years. It should be emphasized at this point that the symptoms produced by gastrinomas do not develop suddenly, but rather in all probability take many years to present the full-blown classic clinical picture. It may well be that a stage of mild to moderate hyperplasia of gastrin-producing islet cells precedes the development of single or multiple adenomas or carcinomas.

Once the syndrome is suspected, the first step is to document the marked increase in basal gastric secretion, which may reach levels of 80 mEq/hour or greater and which fails to increase further with pentagastrin stimulation.

Circulating gastrin. — Normal fasting serum gastrin concentrations are less than 200 pg/ml in man, with an average value in most laboratories approximating 70 pg. Fasting serum gastrin concentrations in patients with a gastrinoma are increased, ranging from 300 up to 350,000 pg/ml.

Intravenous calcium infusion. — In patients with gastrinomas the administration of intravenous calcium (15–20 mg calcium/kg body weight over a period of 3 hours) will produce marked increases in both serum gastrin concentrations and rates of acid secretion. The increases in both acid secretory rates and gastrin levels exceed those observed with calcium infusion in normal patients and in patients with the common variety of duodenal ulcer disease.

In normal individuals and patients with common peptic ulcer disease, feeding a test meal results in increases in serum gastrin concentrations, whereas in patients with gastrinomas there is no significant rise. The absence of a significant postcibal gastrin release in gastrinomas is consistent with the thesis that persistent gastric hyperchlorhydria has suppressed secretion of gastrin by the antral and duodenal mucosa, that the neutralizing effect exerted by the test meal on the acid in the stomachs of these patients is negligible and that the release of gastrin by these tumor cells is not stimulated by the usual secretagogues contained in food.

In resume, the diagnosis of gastrinoma hinges upon (1) a high index of suspicion on the part of the clinician, (2) the demonstration of marked basal gastric acid hypersecretion not increased by pentagastrin or a test meal, (3) the demonstration of marked increase in serum gastrin and (4) further increases with calcium infusion.

Radiologic diagnosis. — The role of the radiologist is to substantiate the severity of the ulcer diathesis by demonstrating multiple upper gastrointestinal ulcers and prominent mucosal folds in the stomach, duodenum and jejunum.

Angiographic demonstration and localization of these tumors is no longer indicated since the diagnosis rests upon the measurement of gastric secretion and serum gastrin, and especially since the only effective treatment is total gastrectomy.

Differential diagnosis. — Patients with pernicious anemia also have high circulating gastrin levels. However, they are achlorhydric.

Gastrin-producing tumors occur throughout the pancreas **(A)** with some predilection for the tail (42%). They are found with almost equal frequency in the body (36%) and less commonly in the head (22%). Approximately 10% are ectopic.

After several years of controversy there is now general agreement that patients with full-blown Zollinger-Ellison syndrome and its complications should undergo a total gastrectomy after histologic confirmation by biopsy and frozen section of the tumor at laparotomy.

Since the full-blown clinical picture may take years to develop and since spontaneous remissions have been reported, laparotomy and total gastrectomy **(B)** should be reserved for patients in whom the symptoms are incapacitating or complications have occurred.

In most patients, especially if they have a narrow angle between the costal margins, a midline incision **(C)** extending from the xiphisternum to 3 cm below the umbilicus will provide the best exposure. In case there is need for additional exposure, the incision in the linea alba can be extended along the left border of the xiphisternum to the costal margin; however, this maneuver may substantially increase or prolong incisional pain, and for this reason should be used only on rare occasions.

Once a cursory general abdominal exploration is accomplished, the next step is to establish a tissue diagnosis of islet cell tumor.

The gastrocolic ligament is divided to enter the lesser peritoneal space and to gain exposure of the body and tail of the pancreas **(D)**.

[Total gastrectomy *continued on page 192.*]

PLATE 41

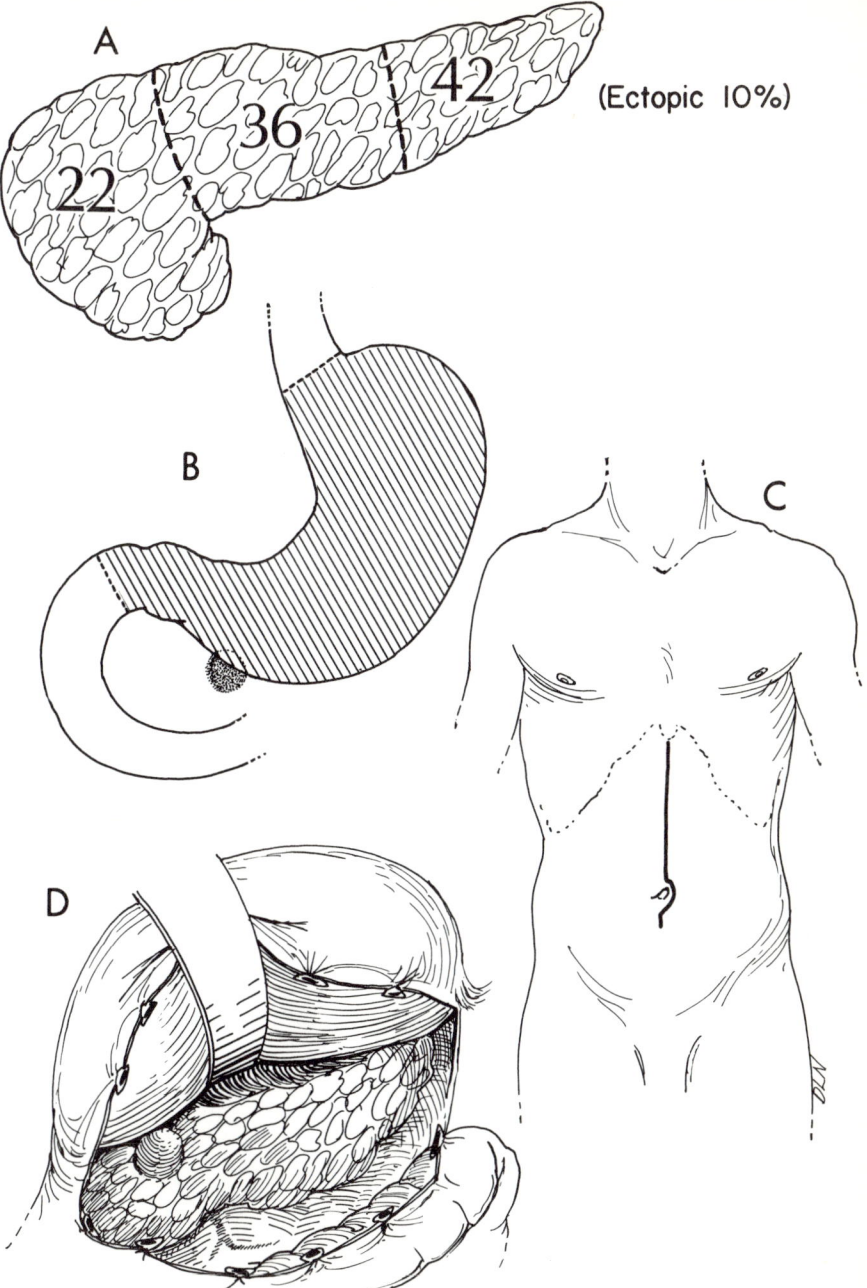

(Ectopic 10%)

The head is exposed by a Kocher maneuver **(E)**. If an enlarged lymph node, potentially containing a metastasis, is located, it is excised for frozen section; if a diagnosis cannot be established in this manner, the technic of incisional biopsy **(F)** for tumors located in the head and body and excisional biopsy for tumors located in the tail is utilized for frozen section. Excisional biopsies of tumors in the head or body increase unnecessarily the risk of pancreatic duct obstruction and the possibility of ensuing and potentially lethal postoperative acute pancreatitis.

Once a tissue diagnosis is established, the surgeon proceeds with a total gastrectomy, which must be ascertained by including a 1-cm cuff of duodenum at the distal end and a few millimeters of whitish squamous esophageal mucosa proximally. Even a small cuff of gastric mucosal remnant may produce gastric hypersecretion with its inherent complications, especially when this remnant is anastomosed to the jejunum, which has a much lower resistance to ulcerations than the duodenal mucosa.

Total gastrectomy begins with the mobilization of the pylorus. Great care is exercised to avoid unnecessary dissection of the head of the pancreas. For purposes of traction a large Penrose drain is passed around the midportion of the stomach. A straight Bainbridge forceps is applied on the duodenum just distal to the pylorus **(G)**. A Payr clamp is placed on the pylorus to avoid spillage of any gastric content that may have not been aspirated by the nasogastric tube.

The duodenum is incised along the Bainbridge clamp. Closure of the duodenal stump begins **(H)**.

[Total gastrectomy *continued on page 194.*]

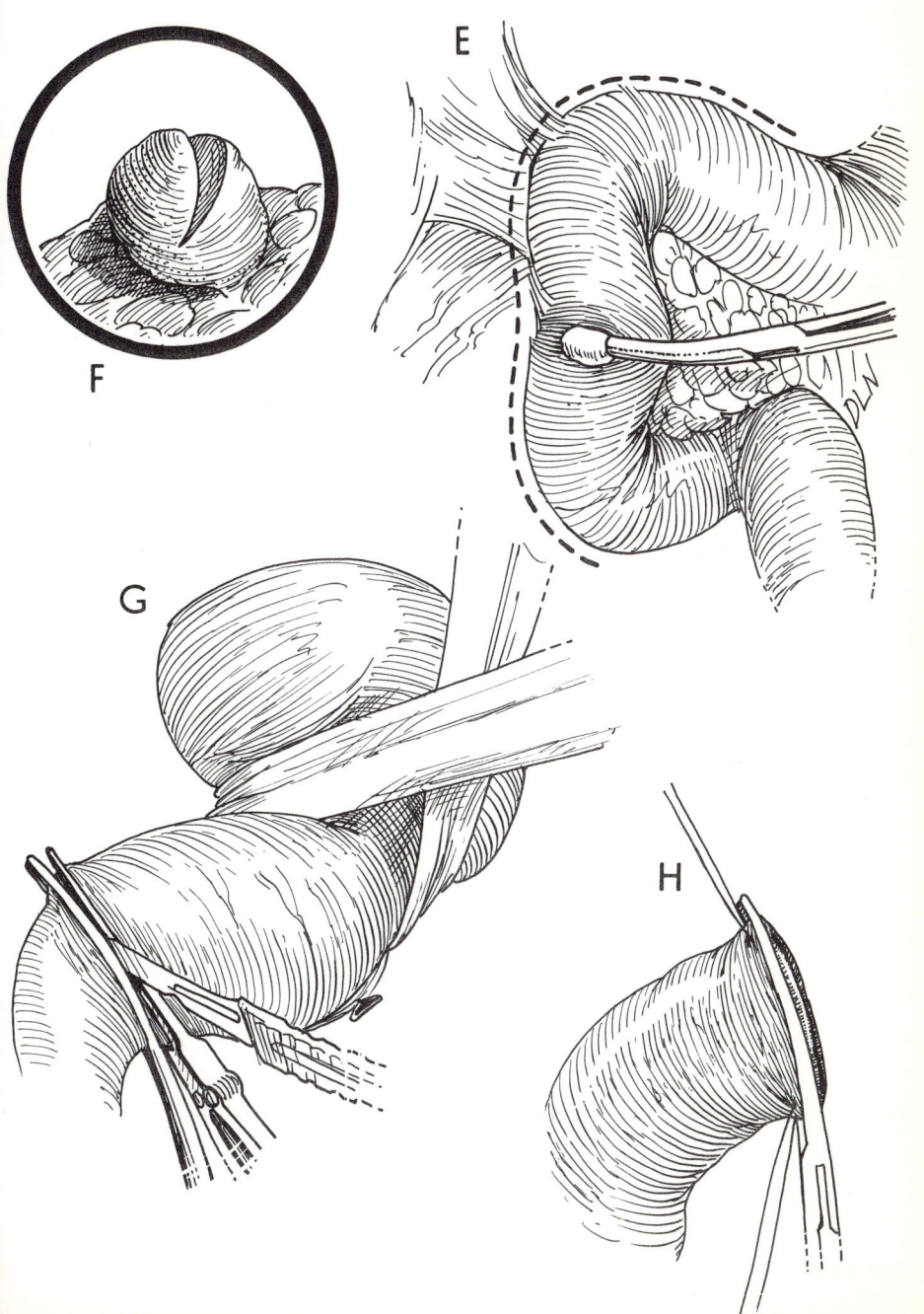

The duodenal stump is closed by the Parker-Kerr method of oversewing a clamp, in 2 layers. The first is a continuous row over the clamp with 00 or 000 chromic catgut **(I)**. Once the entire length of the duodenal stump is loosely sutured the clamp is gradually withdrawn with the point down, in an inverting motion, as tension is applied on the catgut suture. This maneuver should invert the duodenal stump. The stump is oversewn lightly with another row of the same catgut suture. The second row consists of interrupted (Lembert) 0000 nonabsorbable sutures **(J)**. A segment of omentum is loosely sutured over the duodenal stump.

Dissection proceeds along the greater and lesser curvatures of the stomach, after the division of the right and left gastric vessels, the gastroepiploics and short gastric vessels, close to the wall of the stomach **(K)**. Tension on the stomach is maintained during the dissection by the assistant, who applies traction on the Payr clamp and the Penrose drain **(L)**.

Great care is taken to protect the pancreas and spleen during the dissection.

[Total gastrectomy *continued on page 196.*]

PLATE 41

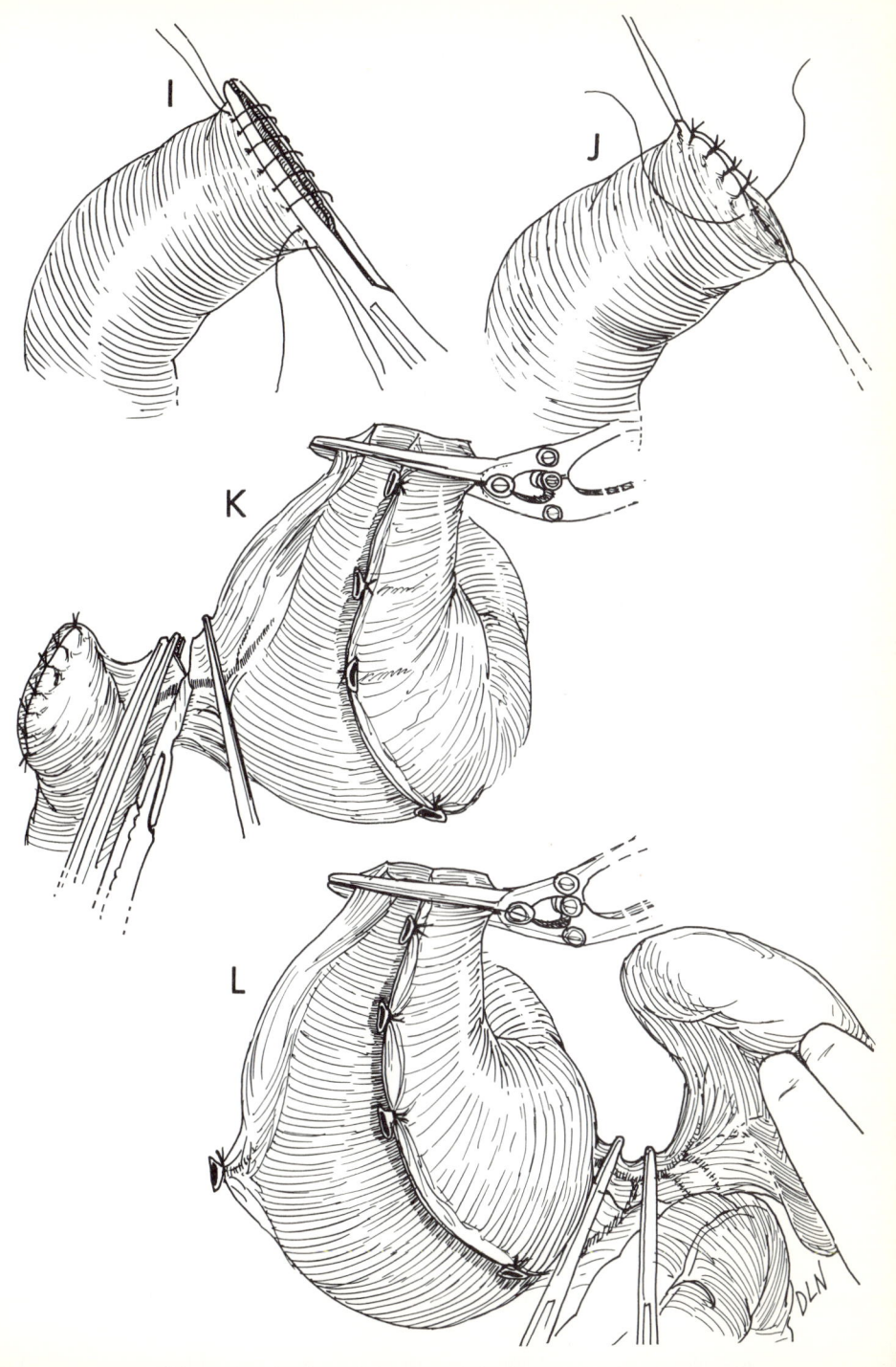

Esophagojejunostomy

While traction is maintained on the stomach, the distal 1.5 cm of esophagus is dissected and mobilized by dividing the 2 vagus trunks between metallic clips **(M)**. The esophagus is dissected and manipulated to a minimal degree to preserve its vascular supply, which will be so important to the integrity of the anastomosis about to be constructed. Clamps should *not* be applied on the esophagus.

Once the distal esophagus is mobilized and while the stomach is still in continuity, the transverse colon is lifted **(N)**, the middle colic vessels identified and a window made in the transverse mesocolon, through which the first loop of the jejunum, just distal to the ligament of Treitz, is passed.

[Esophagojejunostomy *continued on page 198.*]

PLATE 41

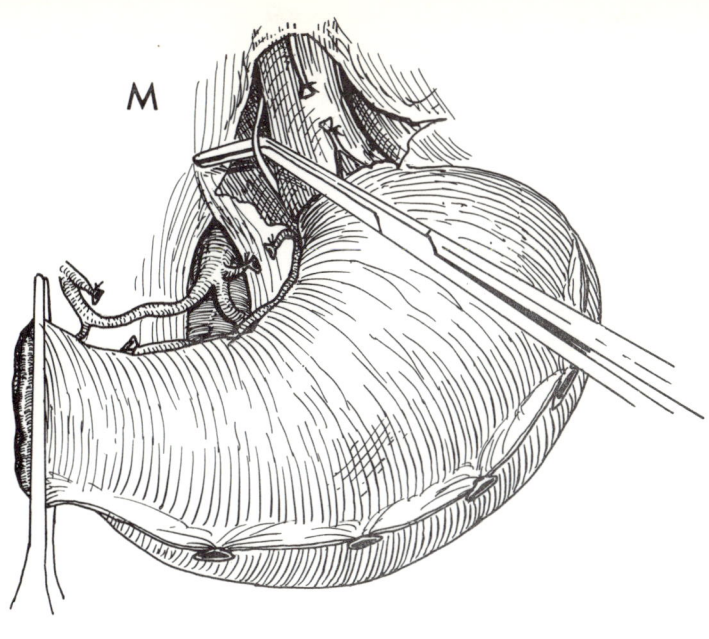

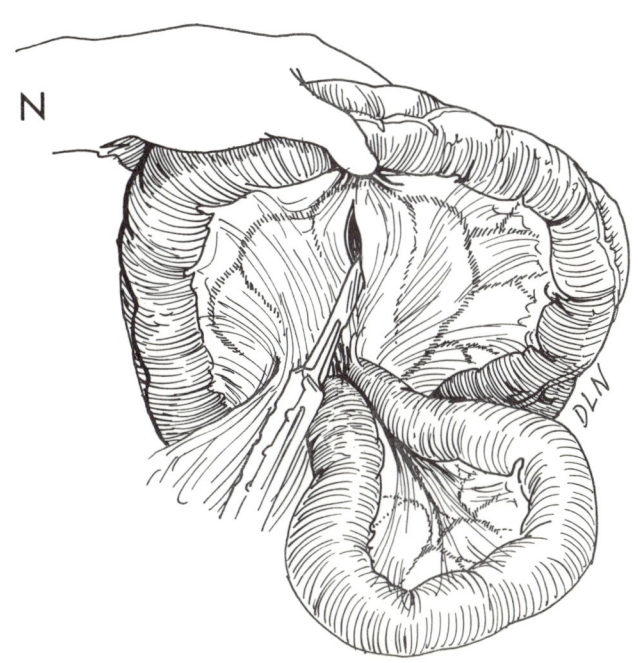

Once the site of anastomosis on the loop of jejunum is chosen, it is juxtaposed to the posterior surface of the esophagus, while the first assistant lifts the stomach (still in continuity with the esophagus) out of the way **(O)**. He maintains tension on the esophagus by applying traction on the stomach, which now serves only as a handle and obviates the use of clamps and stay sutures on the esophagus.

The anastomosis of the end of the esophagus to the side of the jejunum is constructed in 2 layers: (1) an outer row of interrupted Lembert-Cushing stitches utilizing a nonabsorbable 0000 suture: (2) an inner layer of continuous inverting Connell stitch with 000 chromic catgut. Once the posterior side of the outer layer is completed with a row of interrupted 0000 sutures, the esophagus is hemitransected and the jejunum is incised **(P)**.

At this point (with the stomach still in partial continuity with the esophagus) the inner row of continuous catgut suture is completed on the posterior side of the anastomosis.

The nasogastric tube is passed through the anastomosis and guided into the second portion of the duodenum **(Q)**. The inner row of the anastomosis on the anterior side is completed, as the remaining portion of the esophagogastric junction is transected in a stepwise fashion **(R)**.

The outer layer of interrupted sutures is applied on the anterior surface of the anastomosis **(S)**. Great care is taken to assure an adequate lumen.

Since the muscle fibers of the esophagus are parallel to its long axis, the sutures of the outer row are placed perpendicularly (like Cushing stitches) to the muscle fibers and therefore are parallel to the anastomotic line. On the jejunal side the sutures are placed perpendicularly to the anastomotic line, like true Lembert stitches.

[Esophagojejunostomy *continued on page 200.*]

PLATE 41

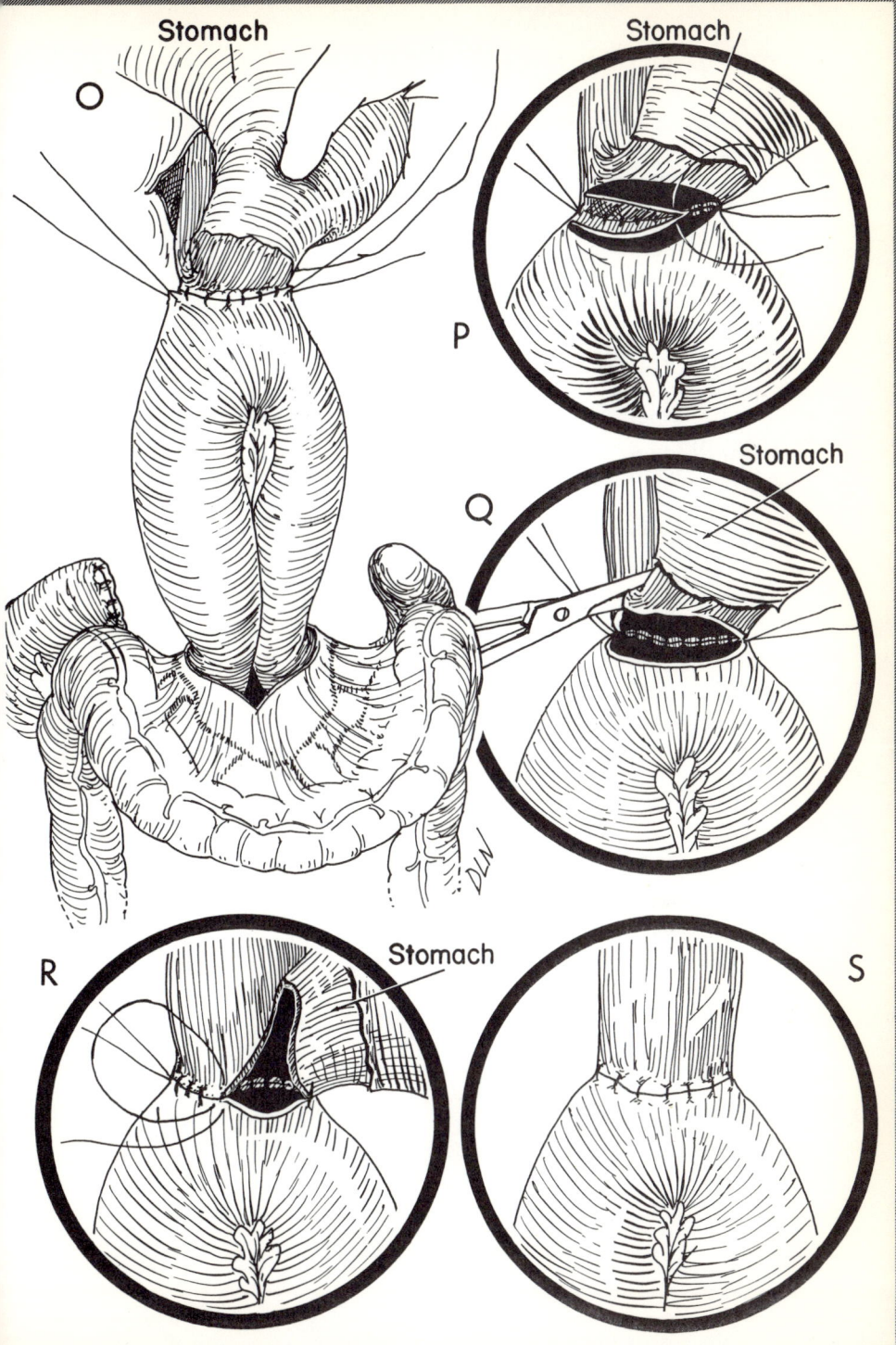

To provide additional support for this anastomosis, the jejunum is sutured with 0000 interrupted stitches to the diaphragm **(T)**.

To divert the duodenal contents away from the esophagus and therefore minimize the changes of alkaline esophagitis, a side-to-side jejunojejunal anastomosis in 2 layers is constructed. Prior to the completion of the jejunojejunal anastomosis, with the lumen of the bowel still open, the position of the nasogastric tube is adjusted to be sure its tip is positioned in the second portion of the duodenum, so that effective drainage of bile and pancreatic juice is assured **(U)**.

The defect in the transverse mesocolon is closed by suturing its edges to the 2 loops of jejunum.

The abdominal cavity is irrigated and the wound is closed **(V)**.

[Alternate method of jejunojejunostomy *on page 202.*]

PLATE 41

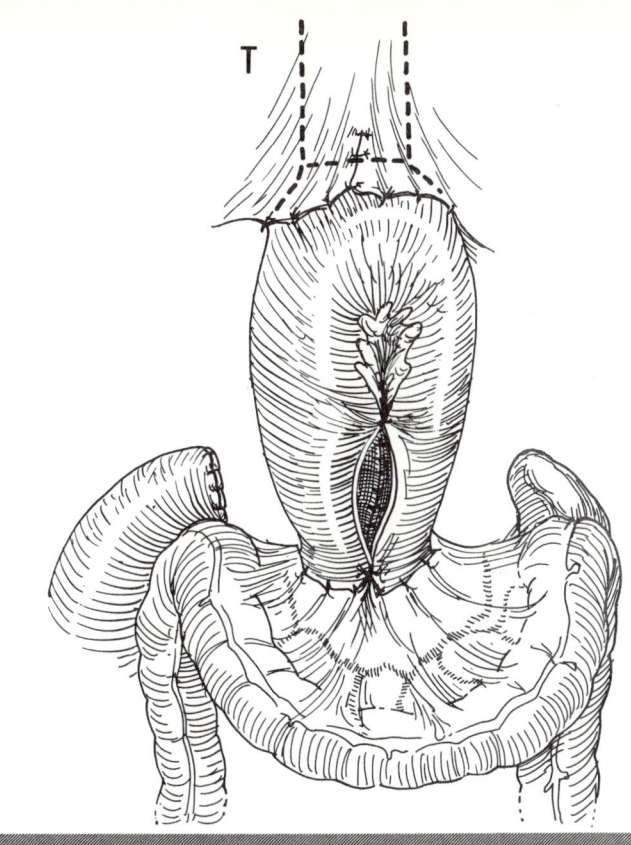

T

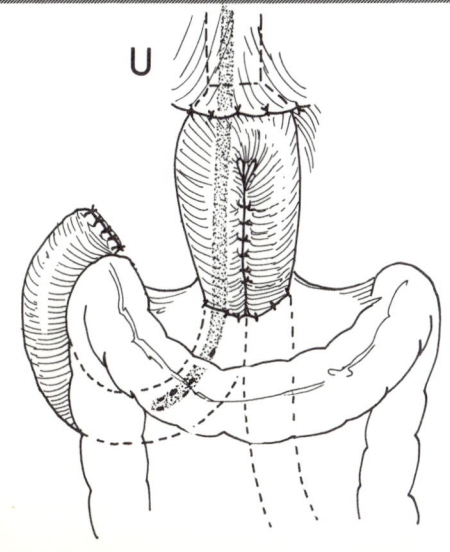

U

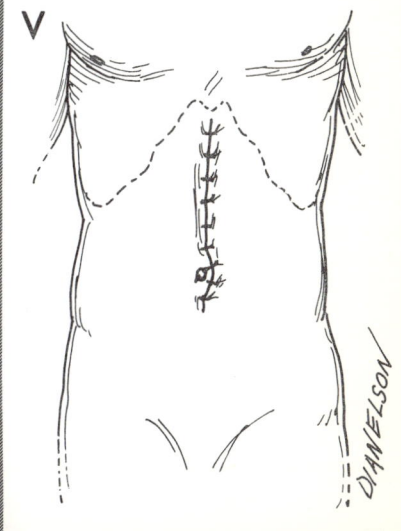

V

There may be some advantage in constructing the jejunojejunal anastomosis beneath the transverse mesocolon **(W−Y)**. This may reduce the chances of alkaline esophagitis by providing a longer segment of jejunum between the esophagus and this anastomosis. Furthermore, the transverse mesocolon may act as a dam.

PLATE 41

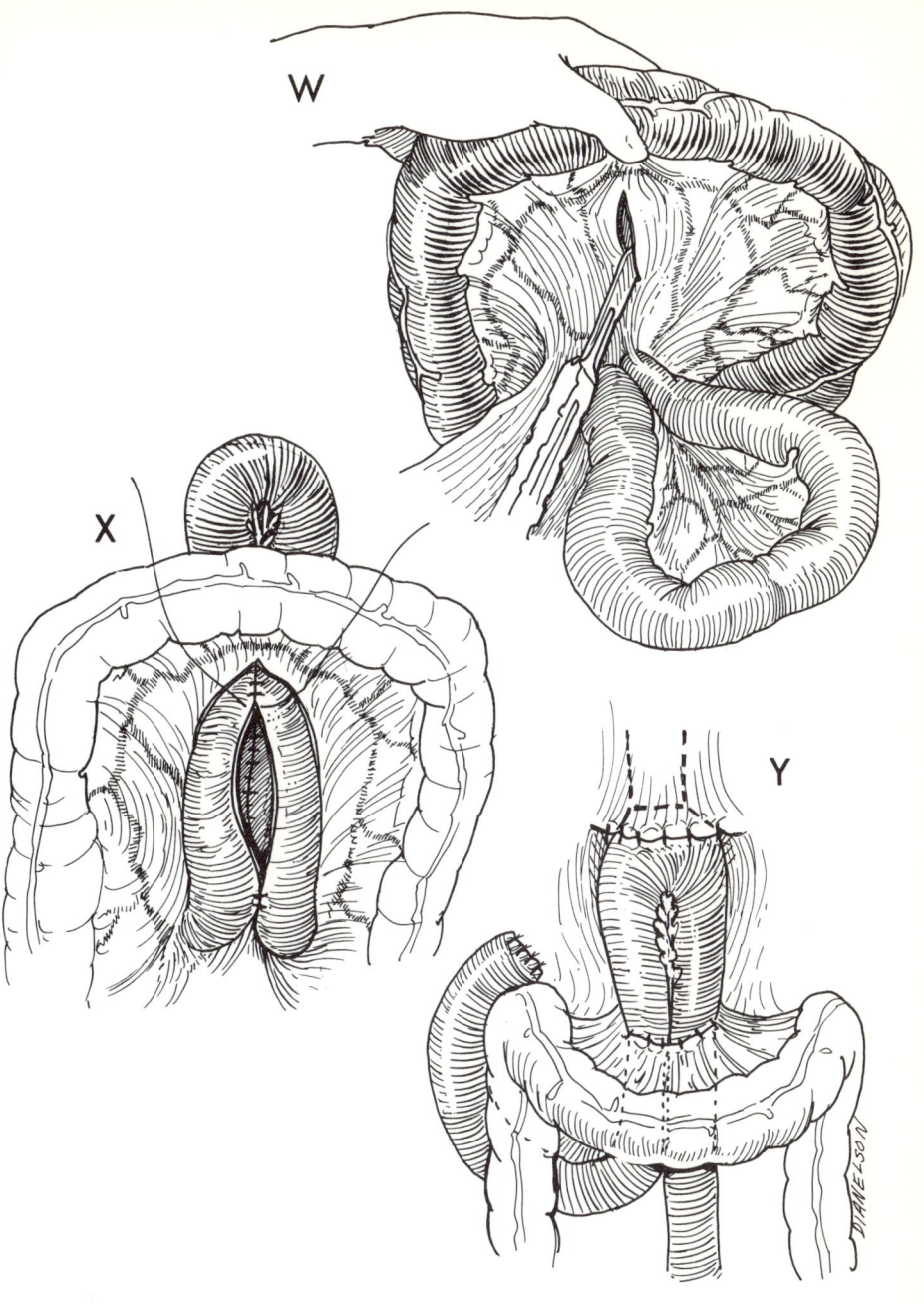

Diarrheogenic Islet Cell Tumors
(Pancreatic Cholera, WDHA Syndrome)

HISTORY.—Verner and Morrison in 1958 described 2 patients with non-beta islet cell tumors of the pancreas who died of the effects of severe refractory watery diarrhea and hypokalemia without any evidence of peptic ulceration. In 1960 Chears and his associates reported a cure of such a patient following resection of a non-beta islet cell tumor. In 1961 Murray and associates demonstrated the absence of acid in 1 such patient, thus establishing a distinction between these patients and those with the Zollinger-Ellison syndrome.

The diarrhea is so severe that it has been characterized as "pancreatic cholera." Later the name of the disease was changed by Marks and co-workers to WDHA syndrome, the acronym denoting the main features of watery diarrhea, hypokalemia and achlorhydria.

There has been a considerable degree of speculation regarding the nature of the humoral mechanisms underlying these clinical features. The hypersecretion of secretin and gastrone, the combined hypersecretion of gastrone and glucagon and the hypersecretion of an enterogastrone known as gastric inhibitory polypeptide have been suggested as possible mechanisms. More recently, high levels of a circulating vasoactive intestinal peptide (VIP) have been reported in these patients and appear to be well correlated with pancreatic islet cell tumors in this syndrome.

CLINICAL FEATURES.—The classic clinical features are explosive watery diarrhea associated with hypokalemic acidosis and low or absent gastric acid secretion, which is histamine-fast. Muscular weakness secondary to the hypokalemia is a prominent feature.

DIAGNOSIS.—The diagnosis is suspected in a patient with the clinical features described above upon finding a low gastric acid secretion or achlorhydria that is histamine-fast. The diagnosis is confirmed by selective celiac and superior mesenteric arteriography, which in most instances demonstrates these highly vascular tumors.

By the time the tumors are suspected and diagnosed today they have reached large proportions, and about 50% have metastasized to the liver. Approximately 64 documented cases have been reported to date. Undoubtedly these numbers will increase with further characterization of the polypeptide(s) responsible for this syndrome and further refinements in specific immunoassays, which will allow the diagnosis in earlier stages.

TREATMENT. — Treatment in the cases diagnosed to date has been highly unsatisfactory since at least 50% of these tumors are metastatic. Resection of the tumor is the treatment of choice.

In recurrent and metastatic disease, none of the chemotherapeutic agents tried thus far have proved effective. X-ray therapy may afford some relief in a few instances.

Glucagonomas

In 1966 McGavran and co-workers documented the first case of glucagon-secreting alpha cell carcinoma of the pancreas. In 1969 hyperglucagonemia was described in the polyglandular adenoma syndrome. A few sporadic glucagonomas have been described since then, usually as part of a polyglandular adenoma syndrome.

There is no distinct clinical syndrome associated with the hypersecretion of glucagon by these tumors, except for the presence of diabetes mellitus in over 50% of patients.

The symptoms are usually those of the associated multiple endocrine adenomas. Treatment is directed at the associated endocrine tumors. In 1 instance the glucagonoma was detected and resected during the course of adrenalectomy for Cushing's syndrome. Recently Mallinson and associates described the disappearance of both diabetes mellitus and a characteristic skin lesion after excision of a glucagonoma.

Resume

To date there are 3 distinct clinical syndromes associated with pancreatic islet cell tumors: (1) insulinomas, associated with hypoglycemia; (2) gastrinomas, with gastric hypersecretion and severe ulcer diathesis; (3) WDHA syndrome, associated with the hypersecretion of an unidentified polypeptide hormone(s). During the next few years we may see the characterization of a fourth clinical syndrome associated with glucagonomas or alpha cell hyperplasia.

CHAPTER 4

The Adrenal Gland

Between 1912 and 1932 Harvey Cushing called attention to the association of basophilic pituitary adenomas and adrenal hyperplasia in patients with the clinical hallmarks of Cushing's syndrome. Because in some partial hypophysectomy effected a return to normal health, Cushing reasoned that hypersecretion of adrenal products caused the striking clinical syndrome. Indeed it was not long after that Cushing's syndrome became recognized in patients without pituitary adenoma. Then it was found that Cushing's syndrome, from whatever cause, was fatal if unresponsive to partial hypophysectomy, because of the ravages of glucocorticoid-accelerated catabolism with striking wasting of tissues and heightened susceptibility to overwhelming infection.

The era of surgical approaches to diseases of the adrenal gland and adrenalectomy for patients with metastatic breast cancer began only when, in 1948, cortisone became available for the management of operatively induced primary adrenal failure or iatrogenic Addison's disease, a fatal condition if left untreated. Operative cures of several adrenal diseases thus became possible

Although glucocorticoid support with cortisone represents an essential need by the organism to withstand stress, disturbances in electrolyte balance in the adrenalectomized patient had to be managed initially by high salt intake or by the parenteral administration of deoxycorticosterone acetate. In 1951 Tait and Simpson successfully isolated aldosterone, the major mineralocorticoid of adrenal gland origin, and this discovery led to the eventual synthesis of an orally effective and potent mineralocorticoid. Thus it became possible to ablate the adrenal glands operatively if necessary and maintain health with oral therapy, recognizing the need to augment glucocorticoid therapy in periods of maximal stress from a maintenance dose of 30 mg to as much as 300 mg cortisone daily.

It is of interest that nature in her infinite wisdom arranged the adrenal gland so that the medullary or catecholamine-secreting portion is wrapped around by the steroid hormone-secreting cortex. Until recently the reason for this nexus was far from obvious, but recent elegant studies have shown that adrenal cortical secretions are essential for the functional integrity of the adrenal medulla. Levels of cortisol found in the systemic circulation are insufficient, however, to maintain adrenal medullary secretion in hypophysectomized animals with adrenal cortical atrophy secondary to the absence of ACTH. Medullary function is repaired in such animals only when levels of cortisol are raised to concentrations approximating that which in fact perfuses the adrenal medulla, as cortical secretions are conveyed centrally through rich sinusoidal venous lacunae within the adrenal medulla toward their egress into the systemic circulation via the central adrenal vein. This understanding may help to explain the occasional simultaneous occurrence of Cushing's disease and pheochromocytoma.

Steroidogenesis and Control of Secretion

Cholesterol is the precursor for all adrenal cortical hormones. The principal corticoids are cortisol (compound F), deoxycorticosterone acetate (DOCA) and aldosterone. Other corticoids, such as androgens and estrogens, are also secreted by the adrenal cortex. Cortisone (cortisol), the hormone of stress, is essential for life. During maximal stress cortisol secretion increases from 30 to 300 mg/day. Aldosterone is the major salt-retaining hormone. In primary adrenal failure, idiopathic or iatrogenic, both glucocorticoid and mineralocorticoid replacement is required. In states of pituitary ACTH deficiency glucocorticoid support alone will suffice.

Control of cortisone secretion is via the stimulatory effect of pituitary ACTH. Secretion of ACTH, which responds quickly to stress situations, is mediated in large part through hormonal signals derived from the central nervous system, probably primarily from the floor of the hypothalamus, from which a rich portal vascular cascade takes origin and flows to the anterior pituitary. Corticotropin-releasing factor (CRF) of central nervous system origin has yet to be isolated and characterized.

Although ACTH is required for the functional anatomy of the outer rim of the adrenal cortex, the zona glomerulosa, it does not play a significant role in maintaining secretion of aldosterone.

Adrenal Gland: Embryology

Of the regulators of aldosterone secretion, sodium and potassium concentrations and ACTH, by far the most important is the renin-angiotensin system. This system is sensitive to changes in plasma volume, as reflected in perfusion through the afferent arteriole of the glomerulus in the region of the juxtaglomerular apparatus, a group of specialized cells that secrete the enzyme renin. This enzyme acts on a plasma α_2-globulin and splits off a decapeptide, angiotensin I, which on passage through the lungs loses 2 amino acids and becomes the active octapeptide, angiotensin II. It is angiotensin II that stimulates adrenal production and secretion of aldosterone, which in turn acts on the distal tubule of the kidney to cause retention of sodium and chloride in exchange for potassium and hydrogen ions.

Embryology

The adrenal cortex is derived from mesoderm; the medulla originates from ectodermal tissue. In some animal species the 2 remain separate. Between the fourth and sixth week of embryonic development, adrenal cortical cells originate from the dorsal abdominal wall near the anterior portion of the mesonephron and condense into larger clusters situated between the root of the mesentery and the genital ridge (A). This developmental origin explains the wide distribution of adrenal ectopic rests as well as the occurrence of estrogenic and androgenic tumors within the adrenal cortex, a result of inclusion of cells from the genital ridge within the cortical primordium.

During the seventh week (11-mm stage), ectodermal neurogenic cells migrate from the neural crest and eventually form the adrenal medulla (B) and other para-aortically situated clusters of chromaffin tissue.

True accessory adrenal glands consisting of cortical and medullary remnants are quite rare and usually occur within the renal cortex or within the celiac plexus. Separate medullary or cortical accessory glands are more frequent. Accessory adrenal cortical tissue with potential for secreting steroid hormones is found in as many as 20% of individuals. Accessory medullary tissue has been found wherever sympathetic ganglion plexuses are located, in the organ of Zuckerkandl near the bifurcation of the aorta as well as in

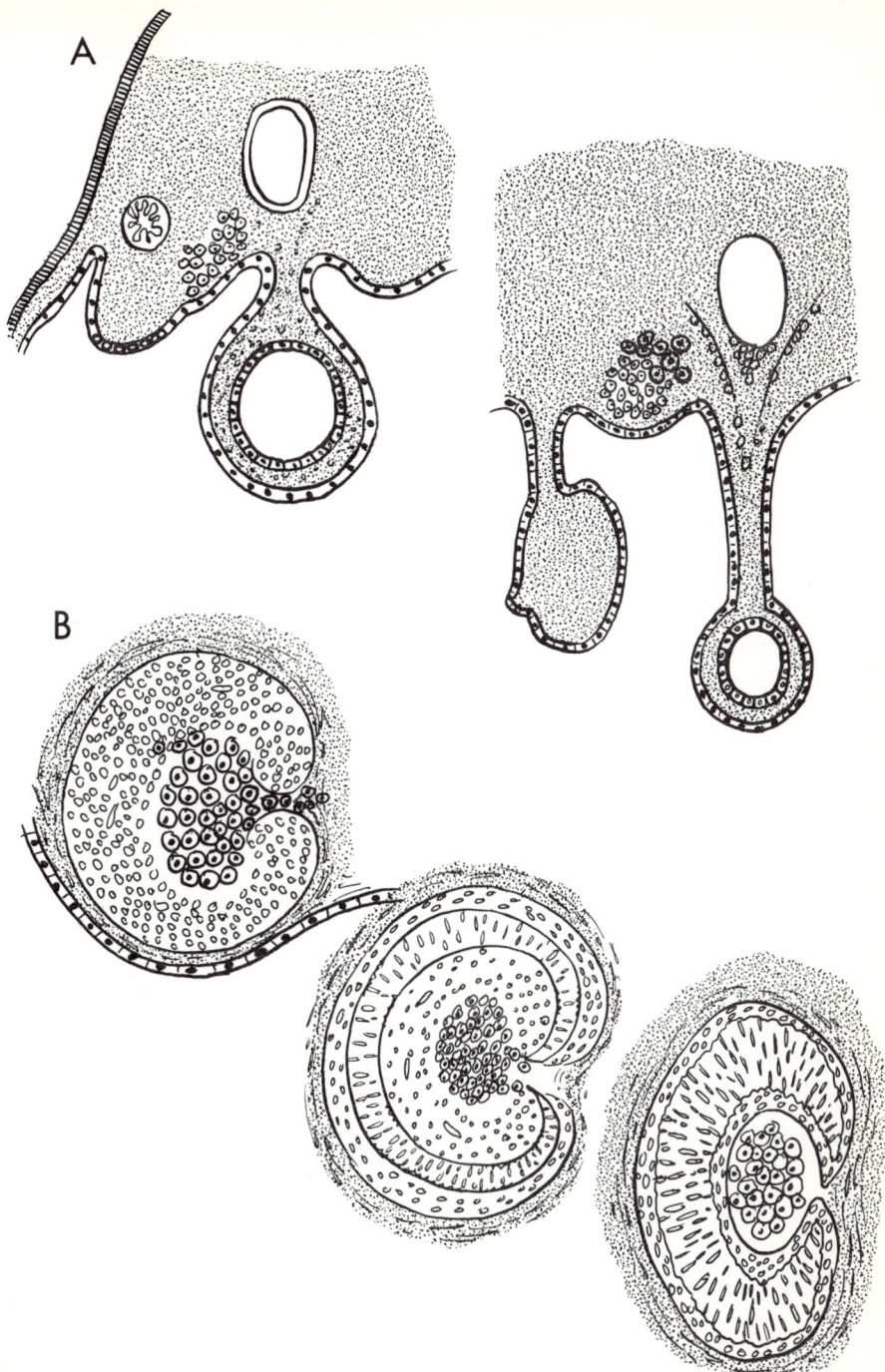

the bladder wall and within the scrotum. There may occasionally be absence of 1 adrenal gland. Bilateral agenesis is extremely rare; it is almost inevitably associated with anencephaly and is invariably fatal in neonatal life.

Anatomy and Histology

The adrenals are triangular caplike structures perched on the superior medial pole of each kidney at the level of the eleventh and twelfth thoracic vertebrae (A). The left adrenal is higher (cephalad) than the right. Adult glands weigh 4-7 gm each and are approximately 30% heavier in males. Each gland is surrounded by fatty tissue within Gerota's fascia. The cortices of the adrenal glands are a golden orange color that contrasts with the pale yellow appearance of surrounding fat.

The rich arterial supply to these glands is mainly derived from the inferior phrenic, the adrenal and the renal arteries (B). This supply is supplemented by branches from the intercostals and the spermatic or ovarian arteries. These vessels pierce the adrenal capsule and branch out into a rich portal circulation that eventually drains into the central adrenal vein. The short right adrenal vein drains directly into the right posterior aspect of the vena cava, and the left adrenal vein, frequently joined by the phrenic vein, empties into the left renal vein.

Light microscopy of the adrenal glands reveals the thin lacy outer zona glomerulosa layer where aldosterone is produced and the major, lipid-rich cortical layers, the zona fasciculata and reticularis, where glucocorticoids are synthesized and secreted. Pituitary ACTH is required for these 2 latter zones. Although ACTH probably plays an insignificant role in the regulation of aldosterone secretion, it is required for glomerulosa cells to respond to trophic stimuli such as angiotensin II.

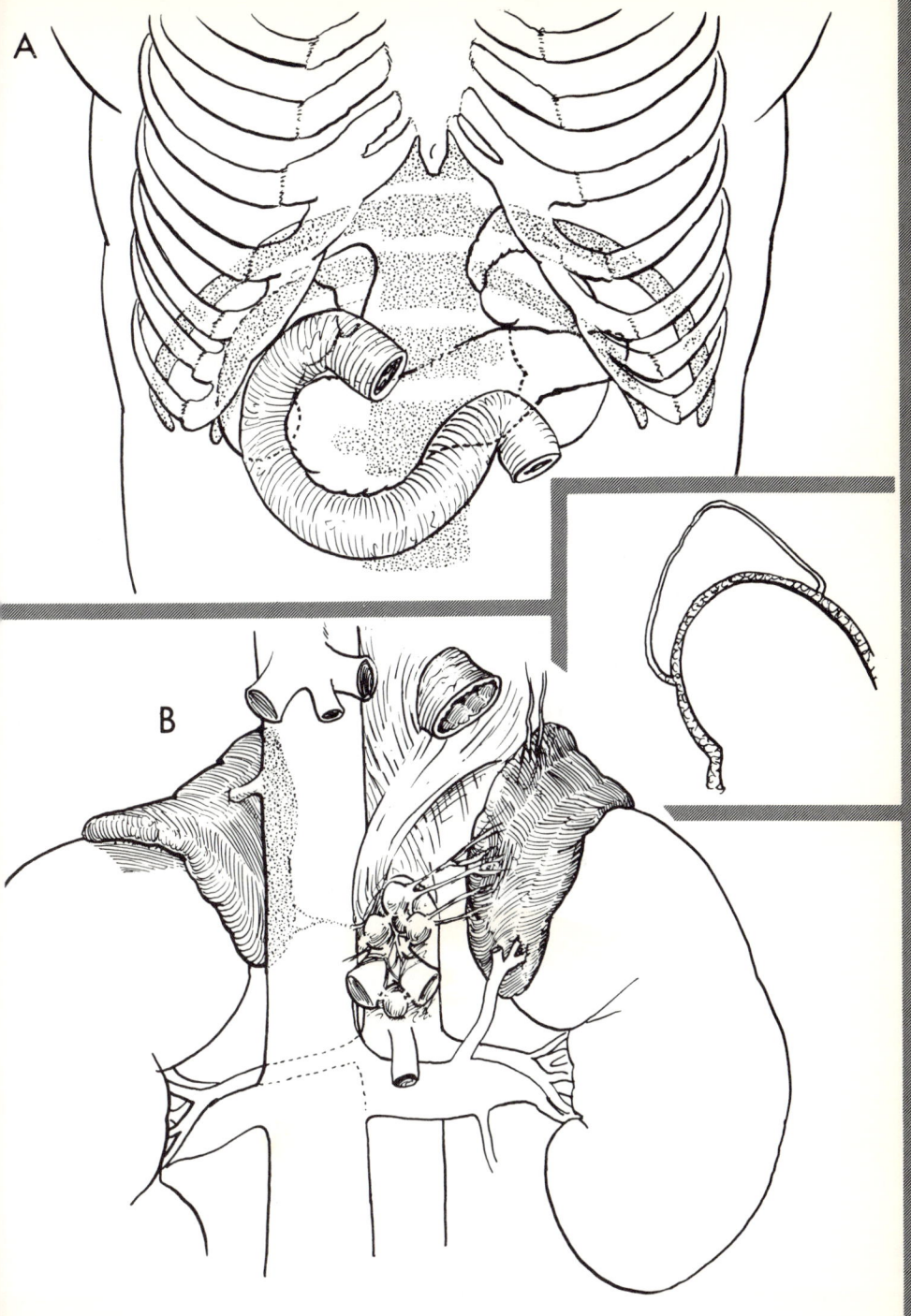

Pathophysiology and Diagnosis of Surgically Managed Diseases

Cushing's Syndrome

Cushing's syndrome is primarily due to excess glucocorticoid secretion. Excessive androgen secretion may also be present, so that the syndrome may be clinically different from patient to patient.

CAUSES.—Cushing's syndrome is in most cases due to bilateral adrenal hyperplasia. Current consensus acknowledges the pituitary dependency of this disease; on occasion a basophile or chromophobe pituitary adenoma may exist, i.e., an enlarged sella turcica is noted. It is speculated that the central nervous system locus of CRF becomes relatively insensitive to the negative feedback effect of prevailing corticoid levels, thus stimulating excess ACTH production, which in turn causes cortical hyperplasia and hypercortisolism.

A corollary to this hypothesis is that on occasion, following bilateral adrenalectomy for Cushing's disease, rapid tumorous growth of the pituitary gland occurs and there is excessive secretion of ACTH and β-MSH. Presumably replacement doses of cortisone are insufficient to exert a normal negative feedback effect upon the central nervous system.

Malignant tumors such as bronchogenic, thymic and pancreatic cancers, among many others, may secrete ectopic ACTH. Usually the clinical manifestations of this form of Cushing's syndrome are mild, but severe hypokalemic myopathy may be striking.

Adrenal adenomas are more commonly seen in children and young adults, but may be encountered at almost any age.

TABLE 4-1.—CAUSES OF CUSHING'S SYNDROME

1. Cushing's disease
   Bilateral adrenal hyperplasia
   Pituitary-dependent Cushing's disease
2. Ectopic ACTH syndrome
3. Adrenal tumor, benign or malignant

CLINICAL MANIFESTATIONS.—These are related to the intense catabolic (tissue-wasting) ravages of excess glucocorticoids (gluconeogenesis) and to the salt-retaining or mineralocorticoid effects of large amounts of circulating glucocorticoids.

DIAGNOSIS.—Establishing the diagnosis of Cushing's disease with certainty may at times prove difficult. Clinical signs and symptoms may be mild, plasma cortisol and urinary 17-hydroxycorticoids may be marginally elevated and urinary 17-ketosteroid values may be normal. In difficult or equivocal cases determination of urinary free cortisol and/or 24-hour cortisol secretory rate may be required as adjunct diagnostic measures.

TABLE 4-2.—CLINICAL MANIFESTATIONS OF CUSHING'S SYNDROME

Ravages of excess gluconeogenesis
  Muscle wasting
  Osteopenia
  Striae
  Poor wound healing
  Excessive bruisability
  Peptic ulcer disease
Mineralocorticoid effects of high levels of cortisol
  Edema
  Hypertension
  Hypokalemia and myopathy
Excess androgens (most prominent in patients with functioning adrenal carcinoma)
  Acne
  Temporal hairline recession
  Hirsutism
  Atrophy of breast tissue
  Clitoral hypertrophy
Other
  Diabetes mellitus
  Leukocytosis
  Psychosis
  Hypercalcemia
  Pancreatitis
  Cholelithiasis
  Renal lithiasis

DIFFERENTIAL DIAGNOSIS. — The dexamethasone suppression test is designed to distinguish the normal from Cushing's syndrome, and pituitary-dependent Cushing's disease from other forms of Cushing's syndrome.

Normally 0.5 mg of dexamethasone every 6 hours will suppress 24-hour urinary 17-hydroxycorticoids to very low levels. In Cushing's disease this dose is almost always insufficient, whereas the substantially larger dose of 2 mg every 6 hours will result in suppression of ACTH secretion and urinary corticoid levels in these patients. Autonomous states of hypercortisolism, such as adenoma or the ectopic ACTH syndrome, are not influenced by high doses of exogenously administered corticoids.

TABLE 4–3. — DIAGNOSIS OF CUSHING'S SYNDROME

Clinical manifestations
Polycythemia, eosinopenia and leukocytosis
Diabetic glucose tolerance test
High plasma cortisol levels with loss of diurnal rhythm (normally high in A.M., low in P.M.)
Failure of 1 mg dexamethasone, administered at bedtime, to suppress 8 A.M. cortisol levels to less than 5 μg/100 ml or 2 mg/day to suppress 24-hour urinary 17-hydroxycorticoids
High 24-hour urinary 17-hydroxycorticoids (greater than 8 mg/24 hours)
High urinary free cortisol
High urinary ketosteroids and/or plasma androgens
Localization procedures (iodocholesterol scan, arteriography, venous angiography)

TABLE 4-4.—DIFFERENTIAL DIAGNOSIS OF CUSHING'S SYNDROME

TEST	HYPERPLASIA	ADENOMA	ECTOPIC ACTH
Dexamethasone suppression*	+	−	−
High 17-KS	+	+++**	+
Increased ACTH	↑ →†	↓	↑
Hypokalemia	±	−	+++
Metyrapone test‡	+	−	−
↑ 17-OH corticoids	+	+	+

*Dexamethasone, a potent synthetic glucocorticoid, is not measured in plasma as cortisol or as urinary 17-hydroxycorticoids. In Cushing's disease, when dexamethasone is given in sufficient quantity (8 mg/day) to suppress release of ACTH, cortisol secretion will drop to low levels.

**Ketosteroid production may be marginally elevated in adrenal hyperplasia, increased where there is an autonomous benign adenoma but strikingly high with a malignant functioning adrenal cortical carcinoma.

†Although adrenal hyperplasia is secondary to ↑ ACTH release, if cortisol secretion is sufficiently high to "please" the disturbed central nervous system locus that regulates ACTH secretion, at any given time circulating levels of ACTH may be normal.

‡When 30 mg/kg of metyrapone is given intravenously over a period of 4 hours, the conversion of 11-deoxycortisol to cortisol is blocked selectively. Normal subjects and patients with cortical hyperplasia will respond with increased secretion of cortisol precursors (measured as urinary 17-hydroxycorticosteroids) as ACTH secretion rises. Patients with adrenal tumors and ectopic ACTH secretion fail to respond.

Cushing's Syndrome

TREATMENT. — Treatment of Cushing's syndrome is dependent on the cause.

1. In Cushing's disease, bilateral adrenalectomy is the most expeditious way to effect an immediate cure. However, some 5–10% of such patients will develop Nelson's syndrome, characterized by hyperpigmentation because of extraordinarily high production of ACTH and β-MSH secondary to rapid growth of the pituitary, which requires aggressive neurosurgery and irradiation.

Because of the central nervous system and pituitary dependency of Cushing's disease, some favor external irradiation to the pituitary alone or in combination with bilateral adrenalectomy. Our own approach is almost always to proceed with bilateral adrenalectomy. If the patient is quite ill because of florid Cushing's disease, then medical therapy with aminoglutethimide, metyrapone, diphenylhydantoin or with ortho, para'-dichlorodiphenyldichloroethane (o,p'-DDD) is instituted for a 2–6-month period before adrenalectomy. This will reduce the heightened operative risks of bilateral adrenalectomy in a patient who has sustained the intense catabolic effects of prolonged cortisol excess. In young persons in whom there is concern for lifelong iatrogenic Addison's disease, autotransplantation of a portion of the hyperplastic cortex into skeletal muscle has been successfully accomplished.

2. Benign adrenal adenomas are resected.

3. The ectopic ACTH syndrome may be temporarily ameliorated if the offending visceral malignancy can be resected. The medical approaches just outlined may be used when operative intervention is inadequate or inadvisable. Adrenalectomy may be indicated as palliative intervention in this syndrome.

4. Adrenocortical carcinomas may be nonfunctioning or may produce features of Cushing's syndrome, virilization or feminization. They metastasize late and grow slowly. If there is no evidence of distant metastases, a re-exploration of the site of excision may be worthwhile. Excision of local recurrences may afford several symptom-free years. Distant metastases appear ordinarily in liver, lungs and bones. Signs and symptoms of hormone excess, which herald recurrences, may be alleviated by the adrenocorticolytic chemotherapeutic agents cited.

INTRAOPERATIVE MANAGEMENT AND SURPRISES. — Cortisone

TABLE 4-5.—TREATMENT OF CUSHING'S SYNDROME

Bilateral adrenal hyperplasia
    Bilateral adrenalectomy with or without autotransplantation
    External irradiation of the pituitary
    Transsphenoidal excision of or insertion of radioactive sources into the pituitary gland
    Medical: o,p-DDD, aminoglutethimide, metyrapone, diphenylhydantoin
Adrenal adenoma
    Resection
Ectopic ACTH syndrome
    Excision, if possible, of the malignant source of excess ACTH
    Medical approaches to excess cortisol production
    Adrenalectomy
Adrenocortical carcinoma
    Excision
    Medical therapy

---

acetate in doses of 200–300 mg daily in divided intramuscular doses every 6 hours should be started on the day of operation. (Intravenous hydrocortisone is *never* the way to manage any patient with inadequate adrenal function). Barring complications, this dose of cortisone can be gradually tapered. Once the daily dose of cortisone acetate is down to 25 mg three times a day, 9α-fluorohydrocortisone (or Florinef), a potent synthetic mineralocorticoid, is begun in a dose of 0.05–0.1 mg daily. There is no excuse for failing to supply this important support for patients who have been deprived of all adrenal function by adrenalectomy. Failure to withstand insensible salt and water loss, especially under warm or hot environmental conditions, will lead ultimately to adrenal crisis in many patients despite maintenance with glucocorticoid therapy.

In adrenal adenoma, where 1 adrenal and a portion of the other remain in situ, it is generally possible to wean the patient from glucocorticoid therapy over the course of 3–9 months.

In the patient with unsuccessfully resected adrenal carcinoma the neoplasm may secrete insufficient amounts of cortisone for life support and the patient may require maintenance therapy with cortisone.

The patient with unsuccessfully treated ectopic ACTH syndrome must receive potassium replacement and close management of acquired diabetes mellitus if and when that problem develops.

[218] *Hyperaldosteronism*

There is a high incidence of cholelithiasis in patients with Cushing's syndrome, and this may not be discovered until laparotomy. Management of the biliary disease is governed by the condition of the patient.

A more ominous and unsuspected surprise is the discovery of severe pancreatitis with widespread fat necrosis. High levels of adrenal corticosteroids have been implicated in the etiology of acute pancreatitis. This operative finding poses a formidable problem; in our opinion, in cases of bilateral adrenal hyperplasia, the right adrenal gland should be excised and the left adrenal exposed and excised through a retroperitoneal approach, if possible, by reflecting the spleen.

Aldosteronism

CAUSES. — Excess aldosterone secretion leads to sodium and water retention and renal wasting of potassium and magnesium. Primary hyperaldosteronism is caused by a single adrenal glomerulosa adenoma, by multinodular hyperplasia or by diffuse hyperplasia of the glomerulosa of the adrenal cortex. An adenoma may be less than 0.5 cm in diameter. Primary hyperaldosteronism occurs twice as frequently in females. Adenomas are almost always unilateral and probably are responsible for 70% or more of cases of primary hyperaldosteronism with hypertension.

Secondary hyperaldosteronism occurs whenever effective plasma volume is low, as in cirrhosis with ascites, the nephrotic syndrome or congestive heart failure, and whenever renal blood supply is compromised, as in long-standing untreated hypertension with benign nephrosclerosis, renal artery stenosis, etc. In each of the latter instances there is augmented renin secretion from the juxtaglomerular apparatus of the kidney. Raised renin levels activate the formation of angiotensin II, a powerful stimulator of aldosteronism. In primary aldosteronism, by contrast, because of aldosterone-induced sodium retention and consequent hypervolemia, renin secretion and renin levels are low. This is a useful differential diagnostic feature that helps to distinguish primary hyperaldosteronism from essential hypertension with benign nephrosclerosis and high renin levels.

CLINICAL MANIFESTATIONS. — The clinical manifestations of primary aldosteronism can be spectacular, with severe hypertension and serious hypokalemia and its attendant complications such as hypokalemic myopathy, hypokalemic nephropathy with inability to conserve water, polyuria and polydipsia. Hypokalemic alkalotic hypomagnesemic tetany can also occur. Usually, however, the clinical signs and symptoms of primary hyperaldosteronism are mild to moderate and are characterized by modest hypertension, inconstant hypokalemic alkalosis, fatigue and polyuria. Acute worsening of the hypokalemia with either kaluretic antihypertensive thiazides or excess salt intake may be the signal that alerts the physician to the possibility of primary hyperaldosteronism.

DIAGNOSIS OF PRIMARY HYPERALDOSTERONISM. — The diagnosis of primary hyperaldosteronism depends on a high index of suspicion, clinical signs and symptoms and careful interpretation of laboratory values and other test results. Abnormally high 24-hour urinary or plasma aldosterone levels in association with low renin levels are strongly suggestive, provided situations are ruled out that would normally promote increased aldosterone secretion (e.g., hypovolemia secondary to diuretics, secondary hyperaldosteronism, salt restriction) or depressed renin secretion (e.g., excess sodium intake with relative hypervolemia, low renin hypertension). Persistent and newly diagnosed high blood pressure associated with clinical signs of hypokalemic alkalosis, high urinary and plasma aldosterone levels and low plasma renin levels despite salt restriction are substantial reasons for recommending exploration.

TABLE 4-6. — CLINICAL MANIFESTATIONS OF HYPERALDOSTERONISM

Hypertension
Hypokalemia (and alkalosis)
  Weakness and myopathy
  Muscle cramps
  Arrhythmias and digitalis intoxication
  ADH-resistant nephropathy with polyuria
  Diabetes mellitus (low potassium levels impede insulin release)
Tetany
  Hypokalemic alkalosis (lowers ionized calcium)
  Hypomagnesemia

Hyperaldosteronism

In many cases in which operative intervention would effect a cure of both the high blood pressure and the hypokalemia, clearcut laboratory values may be difficult to provide. An additional diagnostic ploy is to administer large doses of the drug spironolactone (400 mg/day for 5 weeks), an aldosterone antagonist at the renal tubule. If both the hypokalemia and the high blood pressure are corrected by this therapeutic trial, the likelihood of primary hyperaldosteronism is strong, and surgical resection of an adenoma may result in cure of the hypertension.

From the foregoing it is obvious that the surgeon contemplating adrenal surgery in a patient with suspected primary hyperaldosteronism must work closely with an endocrinologist, whose assessment and opinion will play an important part in the final disposition. Finally, when the diagnosis is essentially certain, iodocholesterol scanning may be of great value in determining the site and size of the problem.

DIFFERENTIAL DIAGNOSIS OF PRIMARY HYPERALDOSTERONISM. — The differential diagnosis of primary hyperaldosteronism deals with the recognition of states of secondary hyperaldosteronism (Table 4–8), the proper interpretation of laboratory results and the differential diagnosis of hypokalemia (Table 4–9).

TABLE 4–7. – DIAGNOSIS OF PRIMARY HYPERALDOSTERONISM

Clinical Manifestations
  Fatigue
  Polyuria
  Polydipsia
  Hypokalemic alkalosis and hypertension in patient receiving liberal salt intake
Laboratory values
  Low plasma renin, despite salt restriction
  High (plasma and/or urine) aldosterone levels, despite salt loading
  Differential venous sampling for plasma aldosterone and renin levels
Localization procedures (iodocholesterol, arteriography, venography)

TABLE 4-8.—DIFFERENTIAL DIAGNOSIS OF HYPERALDOSTERONISM

Primary hyperaldosteronism
Secondary hyperaldosteronism
  Congestive heart failure
  Nephrotic syndrome
  Ascites
  Hypertension with nephrosclerosis
  Pregnancy
  Bartter's syndrome
  Renin-producing tumors

TABLE 4-9.—DIFFERENTIAL DIAGNOSIS OF HYPOKALEMIA

Hyperaldosteronism (primary or secondary)
Other mineralocorticoid excess (iatrogenic or Cushing's syndrome)
Diarrhea, laxative abuse, emesis, villous adenoma of the colon
Licorice ingestion (contains glycyrrhizic acid, which is kaluretic)
Potassium-losing diuretics

TREATMENT OF PRIMARY HYPERALDOSTERONISM.—Treatment of primary hyperaldosteronism is usually operative, but it must be emphasized that this disease can frequently be handled medically. Hypertension will not necessarily disappear with successful excision of a discrete adenoma. Most patients with primary hyperaldosteronism respond to a large dose of spironolactone, 400 mg/day. Operative intervention should not be undertaken unless there is diagnostic certainty. In many patients this would include preoperative demonstration of the adenoma with iodocholesterol scanning. Older patients with a long-standing history of hypertension probably should be managed medically if responsive to spironolactone therapy.

UNUSUAL INTRAOPERATIVE PROBLEMS.—(1) Patients with primary hyperaldosteronism should not be operated upon until depleted body potassium stores are replenished. If patients are not adequately replenished, arrhythmias, tetany, digitalis intoxication and renal failure may complicate the intraoperative course. (2) The aldosterone-secreting tumor may be ectopically located in the ovary, testis, etc. If exploration of the adrenal glands fails to reveal an adenoma, other areas must be carefully examined. (3) Primary hyperaldosteronism may coexist with other endocrine-secreting tumors. (4) Excessive aldosterone secretion from an adenoma may have caused atrophy of normal glomerulosa tissue. With removal of the adenoma a period of mineralocorticoid deficiency may exist and require treatment with 9α-fluorohydrocortisone, 0.05 – 0.1 mg/day.

MASCULINIZING, FEMINIZING AND NONFUNCTIONING TUMORS OF ADRENAL GLAND

CAUSES. — Benign and malignant forms exist. One hundred percent of feminizing adrenal tumors are malignant, despite the gross and microscopic appearance at initial operation. Feminizing and masculinizing adrenal carcinomas or adenomas are rare. Functioning adrenal carcinomas may produce a bizarre spectrum of steroid hormones, causing some masculinizing features and Cushing's syndrome, but with inadequate cortisol production to support life.

CLINICAL FEATURES AND DIAGNOSIS. — Clinical features depend upon the spectrum of biologically active hormones produced by the tumor. Gynecomastia and loss of libido are commonly the first signs of feminizing adrenal carcinoma in men.

Diagnosis is made by laboratory confirmation of abnormally raised hormone levels, together with localization technics, arteriography, venography and iodocholesterol scanning. In differential diagnosis, functioning tumors of gonadal origin must be considered.

TREATMENT. — Resection is the treatment of choice, if this is feasible. The malignant potential of these tumors may not be ascertained at the initial exploration. Radiation treatment to the operative bed seems to help little, but is still used when the situation is grave. Medical treatment with the adrenolytic compounds described earlier has had very little and variable success. Rarely these tumors seem to be ACTH-dependent, and treatment with dexamethasone may slow the progression of the disease. The possibility of adrenal failure due to tumor involvement of both adrenals must be kept in mind and be treated before adrenal crisis develops, especially in nonfunctioning tumors.

Pheochromocytoma and Other Amine-Producing Tumors

The adrenal medulla is a giant sympathetic ganglion. It receives preganglionic fibers directly from the spinal gray matter. These fibers traverse the celiac ganglion without synapsing and enter the adrenal medulla, where they synapse directly with the chromaffin cells that are the equivalent of sympathetic postganglionic fibers. These cells secrete epinephrine and norepinephrine directly into the bloodstream.

Absence of the adrenal medulla is well tolerated by human subjects because of the elaboration of norepinephrine by sympathetic nerve endings, where norepinephrine is synthesized and released in a manner similar to that described for the adrenal medulla. The sympathetic nerve endings do not contain the specific enzyme that converts norepinephrine to epinephrine. In the adult, epinephrine is found only in the adrenal medulla. In young children and infants, epinephrine may be found in the organ of Zuckerkandl, the chromaffin tissue located at the bifurcation of the abdominal aorta.

Functioning tumors of the adrenal medulla (pheochromocytomas) and of other ganglia have fascinated clinicians since the first description of an adrenal medullary tumor by Frankel in 1866, and since the first successful removal of pheochromocytomas in 1926 by Roux in France and Charles Mayo in the United States.

Until recent times the diagnosis and excision of a pheochromocytoma were premiere events; intraoperative and postoperative mortality was high. With the advent of modern methodology to measure catecholamines and their metabolites in urine and in blood, a high degree of diagnostic accuracy has been achieved. With the availability of sensitive cardiovascular monitoring devices and the judicious pre- and intraoperative use of α- and β-adrenergic blocking drugs, the operative challenge has almost been reduced to the routine of an adrenalectomy.

CAUSES. — Pheochromocytomas are of adrenal medullary or sympathetic ganglion origin. Classically they are tumors of the adrenal medulla. They are brownish in color and hemorrhagic by the time they are excised and sectioned in the surgical pathology laboratory. They exhibit the characteristic chromaffin reaction: the development of a yellowish brown color when fixed in a Formalin-potassium bichromate mixture.

Pheochromocytoma

Pheochromocytomas have been called 10% tumors, because approximately 10% are bilateral (Plate 44), 10% occur in extra-adrenal locations and 10% are malignant. Hyperplasia of the adrenal medulla is a new phenomenon that has been noted recently in conjunction with adenomas. In this regard these tumors follow the classic pattern of other endocrine neoplasms, where one may observe the entire pathologic spectrum from hyperplasia to carcinoma. Histologically, it may difficult to classify these tumors as malignant unless distant metastases are seen at exploration.

By the time pheochromocytomas are diagnosed they have usually reached several centimeters in diameter, but they can be as small as 1 cm.

Whereas pheochromocytomas arising in the adrenal medulla usually secrete both epinephrine and norepinephrine, ectopic ganglion chromaffin tumors do not contain N-methyl transferase and are unable to convert norepinephrine to epinephrine. For this reason tumors that secrete a mixture of epinephrine and norepinephrine are usually of adrenal origin, while tumors that secrete norepinephrine exclusively are apt to be situated in extra-adrenal locations.

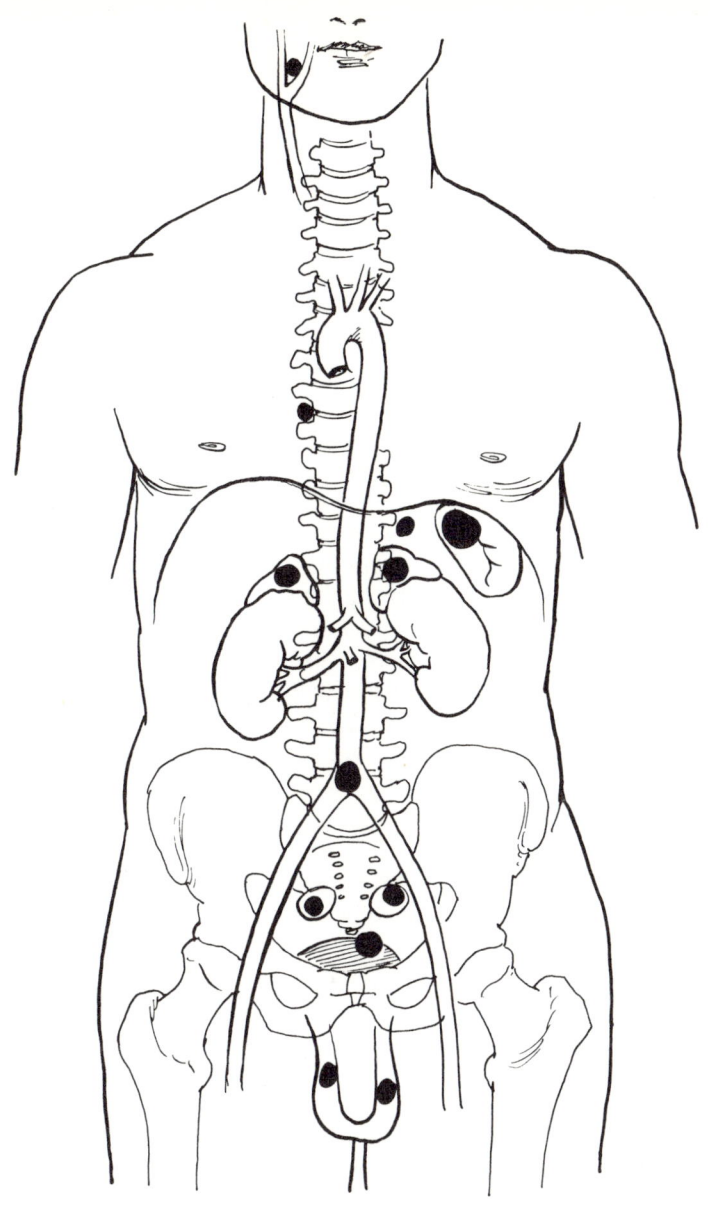

EMBRYOLOGIC DERIVATION OF CHROMAFFIN TUMORS

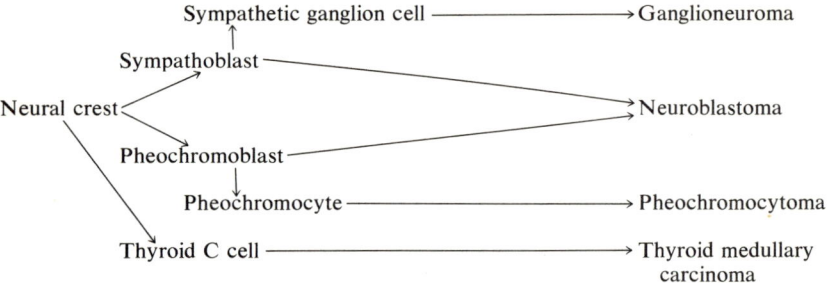

NEUROBLASTOMAS AND GANGLIONEUROMAS. — These arise from the adrenal medulla and other sites of neural crest origin such as the brain, sympathetic ganglia and sympathetic nerve plexuses. Neuroblastomas and ganglioneuromas are found most commonly in the adrenal medulla, but may occur in the retroperitoneal and retropleural spaces and other aberrant sites.

Neuroblastomas are usually large tumors, which occur in neonates and children; they are rare in adults. There may be familial predilection. These tumors arise from sympathoblasts and probably from pheochromoblasts. Local and distant metastases are noted early. Symptoms include diarrhea and occasionally hypertension. The diagnosis is made by the detection of high urinary levels of catecholamine precursors and metabolites such as vanilmandelic acid (VMA), and confirmed preoperatively by radiologic localization technics. Early radical excision, followed by radiation therapy and vigorous chemotherapy, has resulted in "cures," even in the presence of distant metastases.

Ganglioneuromas usually develop during youth, but most become clinically manifest in adulthood. They may become anaplastic and degenerate into malignant neuroblastomas. Unless malignant degeneration has occurred, these tumors do *not* as a rule hypersecrete catecholamine precursors or metabolic products.

Their presence is usually detected by chest x-ray and radiologic localization technics. Operative excision is usually curative. If malignant degeneration has occurred, these tumors are treated as neuroblastomas.

MEDULLARY CANCER OF THE THYROID GLAND. — This tumor is derived from the thyroid C cell, which is of neural crest origin. Ordinarily it secretes calcitonin. On occasion such tumors are the source of excess production of catecholamines; more commonly, however, they coexist with pheochromocytomas. This syndrome has a high genetic penetrance.

CLINICAL FEATURES. — The presenting clinical signs and symptoms reflect the spectrum of biologically active amines secreted from the tumor, its size and whether or not the hypersecretion takes place in paroxysms.

The most heralded feature of pheochromocytoma is the occurrence of paroxysms of hypertension, which are seen in 30–50% of patients. These paroxysms are characterized by extreme hypertension, severe headaches, striking diaphoresis, tachycardia, palpitations, anxiety, a sense of doom and pallor. These symptoms may be accompanied by syncope, nausea, vomiting, angina, visual aberrations, blurred vision and dry mouth. Convulsions have been noted in children. Shock, acute myocardial infarction or cerebrovascular accidents may supervene. The paroxysms may be precipitated by a variety of stimuli such as stress, exercise, stimulation or massage of the tumor, and micturation when the tumor is adherent to the wall of the bladder.

In a substantial number of patients, however, such paroxysms are absent and a symptomatic sustained hypertension may be the only sign.

TABLE 4–10. — CLINICAL MANIFESTATIONS OF PHEOCHROMOCYTOMA

Persistent hypertension 70%	
Paroxysmal hypertension 30%	
Other	
Diaphoresis	Hyperglycemia
Pallor	Hypermetabolism
Tremor	Leukocytosis
Arrhythmias	Ulcer disease
Anxiety	Myocarditis
Headache	Orthostatic hypotension
Nausea	Epigastric pain
Dilated pupils	Angina
Myocardial infarct	Cerebrovascular accident

Other chromaffin tumors, such as neuroblastomas, seldom produce signs associated with an excess of biologically active amines. Hypertension is rarely encountered. A palpated mass, localized gastrointestinal disturbances or anorexia and weight loss associated with metastatic disease may be the initial presenting features.

SYNTHESIS AND DEGRADATION OF CATECHOLAMINES. — The clinical manifestations of pheochromocytomas are caused by excess secretion of catecholamines. The diagnosis of pheochromocytoma rests upon the measurement of these amines and their degradation products in the circulation and in urine. The synthesis and degradation of these amines are outlined here.

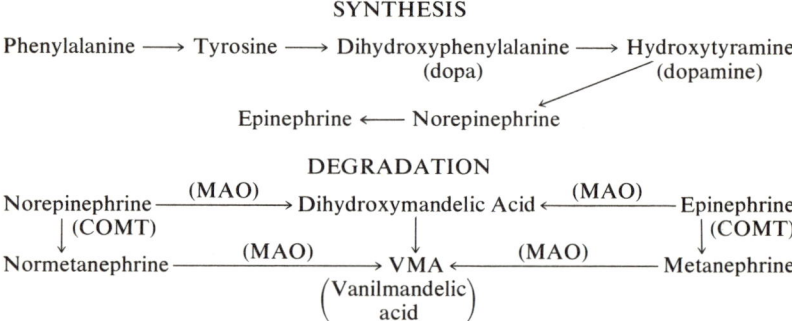

DIAGNOSIS. — In the final analysis, the diagnosis of the presence of a pheochromocytoma or other neural crest tumor is based on laboratory documentation of excess amine production. Measurement of urinary catecholamines may reveal abnormal elevations or, barring this finding, metabolic by-products may be higher than normal. The latter include the metabolites of norepinephrine and epinephrine, the metanephrines and VMA. Metanephrines are formed by the action of catechol-O-methyltransferase (COMT) on circulating catechols, while metabolism within tissue may depend upon oxidative deamination.

TABLE 4-11.—EFFECTS OF ADRENERGIC STIMULATION

	ALPHA	BETA
Metabolic		
Hyperglycemia (glycogenolysis)	—	+
Hyperlipidemia (lipolysis)	—	+
Glucagon secretion	—	Stimulation
Insulin secretion	Inhibition	—
Cutaneous		
Sweat glands	Secretion	—
Pilomotor muscles	Contraction	—
Gastrointestinal		
Motility	Decrease	Decrease
Sphincters	Contraction	—
Pulmonary		
Bronchial musculature	—	Dilatation
Cardiac		
Rate	—	Increase, arrhythmias
Atria and ventricles	—	Increase contractility and irritability
Peripheral vascular		
Skin	Constriction	—
Cerebral	Constriction	—
Coronary and pulmonary	Constriction	Dilatation
Pupils		Dilatation

TABLE 4-12.—DIAGNOSIS OF PHEOCHROMOCYTOMA

High index of suspicion
Increased urinary amines
Total catecholamines > 100 μg/24 hr
Norepinephrine > 70 μg/24 hr
Epinephrine > 20 μg/24 hr
Vanilmandelic acid > 6-7 mg/24 hr
Metanephrine and normetanephrine > 1.3 mg/24 hr
Increased plasma catecholamines (especially useful for selective venous sampling)
Provocative tests (histamine and/or glucagon)

Since the laboratory diagnosis of pheochromocytoma is 97% accurate, there is seldom need to use provocative tests with glucagon and histamine, which provoke hypertension in normotensive patients, or α-blockers such as phentolamine, which lower blood pressure in hypertensive patients.

In the presence of large amounts of urinary VMA in a normotensive patient, the diagnosis is probably neuroblastoma.

TREATMENT.—Excision of these tumors can cure the disease. Both adrenals and aberrant sites must be examined.

Whenever possible, pheochromocytoma patients are medically prepared for operation for at least 2 weeks. Therapy is aimed at control of excessive α- and β-adrenergic activity. Such therapy should be under way prior to any invasive diagnostic procedures as well.

Phenoxybenzamine, a potent α-adrenergic blocker, is administered orally every 6 hours. It is started at a total dose of 10 mg/day and increased progressively until control of blood pressure or paroxysms of hypertension is achieved. The peak effect occurs approximately 2 hours after oral administration. The half-life of blockade is approximately 24 hours, but the effect of daily adminis-

TABLE 4-13.—MEDICAL TREATMENT OF PHEOCHROMOCYTOMA

Alpha-adrenergic blockade
  Hypertension
  Contracted blood volume
Beta-adrenergic blockade
  Tachycardia
  Arrhythmia

tration is cumulative over 3-5 days. Doses as high as 100 mg/day have been required. Rarely phenoxybenzamine is without effect, either because of inadequate absorption or because serious side effects are encountered, such as nausea and vomiting and central nervous system obtundation. Caution must be exercised in glaucoma patients. To avoid hypotension and to ensure response to sympathomimetic pressor drugs after removal of the pheochromocytoma, the last dose of phenoxybenzamine is administered 10 hours before operation is scheduled.

Phentolamine, a parenterally administered α-adrenergic blocker, is used (intramuscular injection, intravenous drip or bolus) when (1) phenoxybenzamine is without effect, (2) in crisis situations, alone or in combination with phenoxybenzamine, and (3) during operation whenever there is a significant rise in the blood pressure and during the manipulation of the tumor. Phentolamine exhibits a rapid but transient effect with onset of action within 30 seconds and duration no longer than 60 minutes after intravenous administration. It is administered at a dose of 5-10 mg intramuscularly every 4 hours preoperatively when phenoxybenzamine is without effect, as a 50-100 mg/L intravenous drip or as a 5-mg rapid intravenous bolus.

Propranolol, a derivative of isoproterenol, an orally effective β-adrenergic blocker, is used preoperatively in doses of 10-40 mg 4 times a day if there is need to control excessive heart rate or arrhythmias. During operation propranolol can be administered intravenously for such problems. Extreme caution must be used when there is a history of asthma or when real or imminent congestive heart failure is at hand. Beta-adrenergic blockade antagonizes normal adrenergic bronchodilation and is negatively inotropic.

Blood volume determinations should routinely be performed to detect the occasional patient with severely contracted blood volume. This will alert the operating team to the probable need to replace plasma over and above estimated blood loss at the time of operation. However, this condition is usually corrected by the preoperative preparation with phenoxybenzamine.

Anesthesia requirements are as would be expected. Scopolamine is used in preference to atropine. There is no contraindication to the use of opiates. Phenothiazines are contraindicated. Induction is not carried out until the patient is more than adequately monitored for blood pressure, pulse, central venous pressure and urine output; α- and β-adrenergic blockers and pressor agents for parenteral administration must be on hand. A critical factor is the background and experience of the anesthesiologist. It is not unusual to witness a hypertensive crisis during the short-lived hypoxia of induction and during manipulation of the tumor; intravenous administration of phentolamine is required for such periods.

Once the last vein is ligated, hypotension may supervene. This is treated with fluid and plasma and, when necessary, with norepinephrine (1 mg/L) delivered into a large central-high-flow vein as a drip.

POSTOPERATIVE MANAGEMENT. — Within 48 hours the patient is detached from the various catheters and monitors. Postural hypotension may signal either hypovolemia and/or adrenal insufficiency; although only 1 adrenal may have been removed, manipulation of the remaining gland can hamper its optimal function for several days.

SPECIAL CIRCUMSTANCES. — *Pheochromocytoma during pregnancy.* — The first indication of the presence of pheochromocytoma may be during pregnancy, when it must be differentiated from toxemia and preeclampsia. The risks of fetal death (stillbirth) or maternal death during labor and the postpartum period are markedly enhanced if the diagnosis of pheochromocytoma is overlooked.

If diagnosis is made during the first trimester of pregnancy, the patient should be managed as if pregnancy did not exist; removal of the tumor may be followed by spontaneous abortion.

During the last trimester, especially near term, α- and if necessary β-adrenergic blockade is instituted for a period of 2 weeks or longer, and simultaneous excision of the tumor and cesarean delivery are planned. This is probably the only approach that assures the greatest chance of maternal and fetal survival.

Bilateral pheochromocytomas. — The accepted treatment for these patients, who constitute up to 15% of the cases reported, has been bilateral adrenalectomy with appropriate preoperative, intraoperative and postoperative gluco- and mineralocorticoid replacement. Adrenal cortical insufficiency is an undesirable by-product of the treatment of these patients. It is hoped that with the perfection of autotransplantation technics this can be avoided in the future.

Malignant pheochromocytomas.—Approximately 10% of pheochromocytomas are malignant. With the advent of long-acting α-blockers these patients' symptoms can be controlled with relative simplicity, especially if the patients are able to tolerate the side effects of the doses of phenoxybenzamine they require. Tumor growth is usually very slow. The authors have a patient who has had miliary hepatic metastases for 25 years, during which time she has raised a family. If phenoxybenzamine is ineffective, α-methyl tyrosine (an inhibitor of tyrosine hydroxylase) may be used. Unfortunately, α-methyl tyrosine produces a syndrome similar to parkinsonism.

Associated medullary thyroid cancer.—Patients with bilateral pheochromocytomas should be screened for associated medullary thyroid carcinoma and hyperparathyroidism (Sipple's syndrome). Conversely, patients with medullary thyroid cancer should be screened for pheochromocytoma, especially if an operation is planned. In the presence of a pheochromocytoma, the treatment of the medullary cancer should be postponed until after the pheochromocytoma(s) has been excised.

In borderline situations, in which catecholamine levels are slightly elevated with no other evidence of a pheochromocytoma, the medullary cancer may well be responsible for the hypersecretion of catecholamines. In these situations a 2-week course of α-adrenergic blockade should precede thyroidectomy in the event a pheochromocytoma has been overlooked.

Pheochromocytoma in children.—Hypertension and hypertensive crisis may be particularly severe in childhood, with rapid progression to congestive heart failure and encephalopathy.

Children are more apt to have bilateral, multiple and extra-adrenal tumors. Both intra- and extra-adrenal tumors may coexist; as many as 6 extra-adrenal tumors have been reported in the same patient. Indeed, the single most important cause of postoperative death in children after the excision of a pheochromocytoma is the presence of an unsuspected additional tumor.

In view of the high incidence of aberrance (30%) and multiplicity (35%), preoperative radiographic localization studies after the administration of α-adrenergic blockers for 2 weeks are essential in children.

Operative Approaches to the Adrenal Glands

There is a considerable degree of disagreement in the literature as to the best surgical approach to the adrenals. This largely stems from the differing backgrounds, training and interests of the surgeons involved, be they urologists, general or endocrine surgeons. The relatively high incidence of bilateral and ectopic pheochromocytomas mandates the abdominal transperitoneal approach.

There are essentially 3 approaches to the adrenals: (1) abdominal transperitoneal; (2) posterior thoracolumbar, and (3) bilateral flank.

In rare instances of massive tumors, the abdominal incision may be extended into the thorax; this has to be planned before the abdominal incision is made. Only 2 of the approaches enumerated are commonly used. For these reasons, the discussion that follows dwells principally on the abdominal and the posterior thoracolumbar routes.

ANATOMIC CONSIDERATIONS

The adrenal glands are tucked away neatly in the retroperitoneal space within the perirenal fat, in close proximity to the vena cava on the right, to the aorta on the left and to the renal vessels bilaterally.

The 3 adrenal arteries (branches of the inferior phrenic and renal arteries and of the aorta) are minute and seldom visualized with clarity during dissection.

The adrenal vein is a large structure, which must be ligated or clipped. The right adrenal vein is usually single; it is best visualized by medial retraction of the vena cava.

On the left, the adrenal vein has 3 large tributaries that course over the anteromedial aspect of the gland for a short distance. It is preferable to ligate the left adrenal vein a good distance from this trifurcation. In the presence of large adrenal tumors there is a marked proliferation of the vascular supply and drainage of the adrenal gland. There may be several adrenal veins that enter the vena cava or left renal vein.

The lymphatic drainage of the adrenal glands arises from a subcapsular plexus and from a separate plexus in the medulla. These lymphatic channels follow the blood vessels of the gland, predominantly of the suprarenal vein, and end in the upper lumbar lymph nodes.

The adrenal glands are provided with many fine nerves that stream toward them from the celiac plexus and the greater splanchnic and enter the glands from the rostromedial aspect. These are principally medullated, preganglionic neurons, which end on the secretory cells of the medulla. They are tough bands that require ligation and sharp dissection. There appears to be only a vasomotor supply to the cortex.

[Abdominal transperitoneal approach to right adrenal *on page 236.*]

Abdominal Transperitoneal Approach to Right Adrenal

The bilateral subcostal or "bucket-handle" incision is preferable, especially in patients who are debilitated and may develop wound problems (A). In a thin patient with a narrow chest and a sharp costoxiphisternal angle, a midline incision through the linea alba may be more suitable.

The incision is made, the peritoneum incised, the clear plastic wound protector inserted and the abdominal structures examined.

The right lobe of the liver is retracted laterally and rostrally with a Harrington retractor (B). The assistant retracts the duodenum medially with a laparotomy pad; these maneuvers expose the superior pole of the kidney.

The hepatorenal ligament, a transparent fold with a sharp edge, is incised; this provides further exposure of the superior pole of the kidney.

The posterior parietal peritoneum at the rostral and lateral surfaces of the kidney is incised. The renal fascia (Gerota's) is entered; this permits retraction of the kidney caudally. This maneuver results in exposure of the right adrenal, which is then pulled out of the retrocaval adrenal fossa. Mobilization of the duodenum by a Kocher maneuver may be necessary in the dissection of large tumors.

The hepatocaval fold of the posterior peritoneum is incised; rarely this may harbor large veins that must be ligated. The dissection of the posterior parietal peritoneum is then continued along the lateral border of the vena cava (interrupted vertical lines in B).

The vena cava is retracted medially with a vein retractor or a cotton pledget; great care is taken not to interrupt caval blood flow. The entire adrenal is now exposed (C). With minimal dissection at the caval border, the large adrenal vein is exposed, dissected and doubly clipped and divided. Supernumerary veins are handled in similar fashion. With caudad traction, the nerve bundles at the medial superior border are exposed and divided. Dissection is completed; the gland is delivered intact (D).

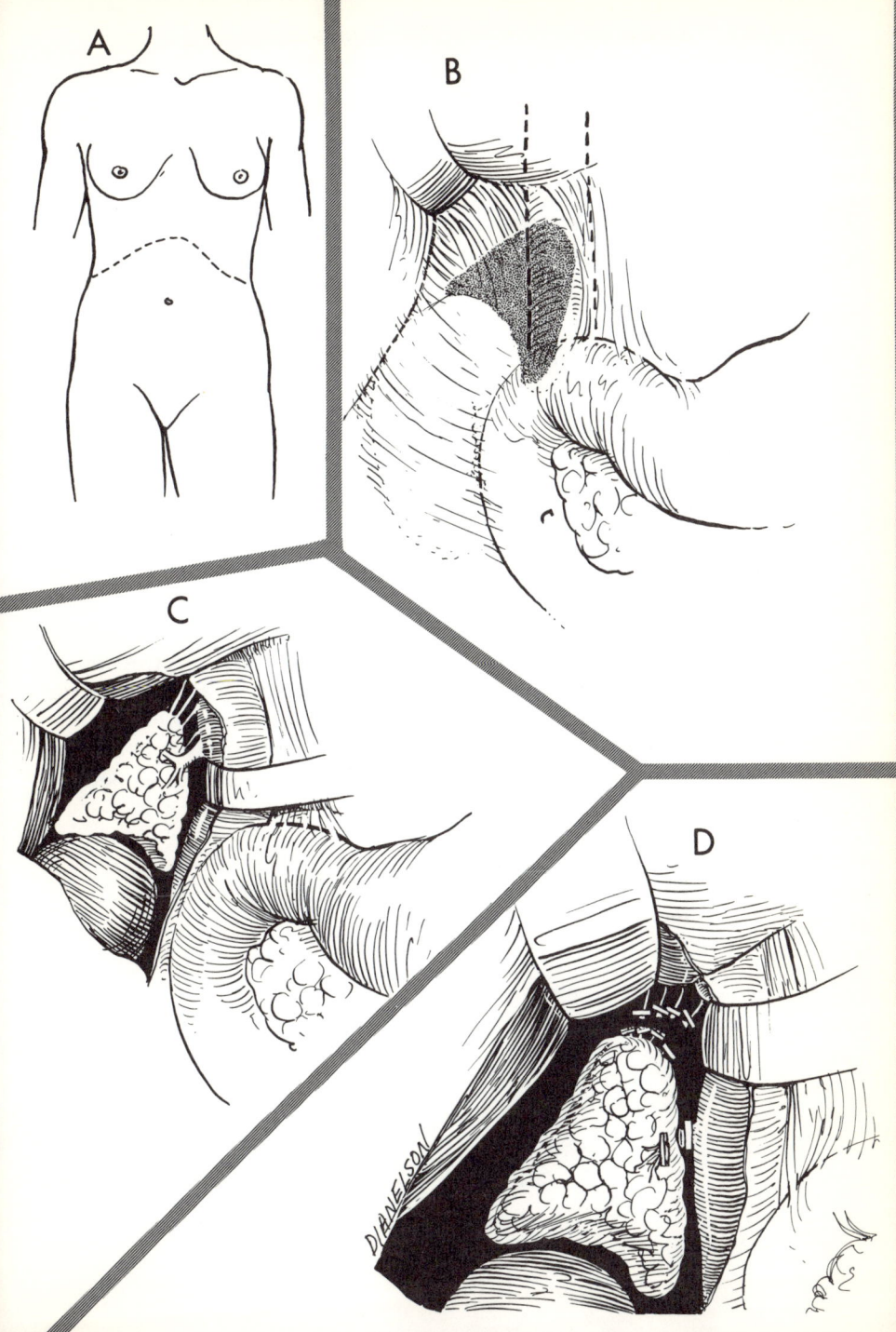

PLATE 45

ABDOMINAL TRANSPERITONEAL APPROACH TO LEFT ADRENAL

The left adrenal gland can be exposed by 2 methods: (1) reflection of the spleen; (2) elevation of the pancreas.

Reflection of the spleen is usually preferable, as it provides excellent exposure of the left adrenal, its hilus and its relationship to the renal vein. In the event the splenic capsule is torn, a splenectomy is performed. The pancreas must be minimally manipulated. With the second method, considerable manipulation and traction of the pancreas is inevitable. Avoiding unnecessary manipulation of the pancreas is of particular importance in Cushing's syndrome, where the incidence of spontaneous pancreatitis (occasionally a surprise finding at operation) is high. Manipulation of the pancreas sets the stage for the development of postoperative acute pancreatitis, with its high morbidity and mortality rate.

REFLECTION OF THE SPLEEN. — The surgeon grasps the spleen and retracts it medially **(A)**. The spleen is covered with a laparotomy pad and held in gentle traction with the left hand. The costal margin is retracted by an assistant with a body-wall (Mayo) retractor. A laparotomy pad is used by the first assistant to retract the splenic flexure of the colon caudally, where it is held in place with the left hand. The splenorenal ligament, now well exposed, is divided **(B)**. The dissection proceeds rostrally until the lienophrenic ligament is divided.

[Approach by reflection of the spleen *continued on page 240.*]

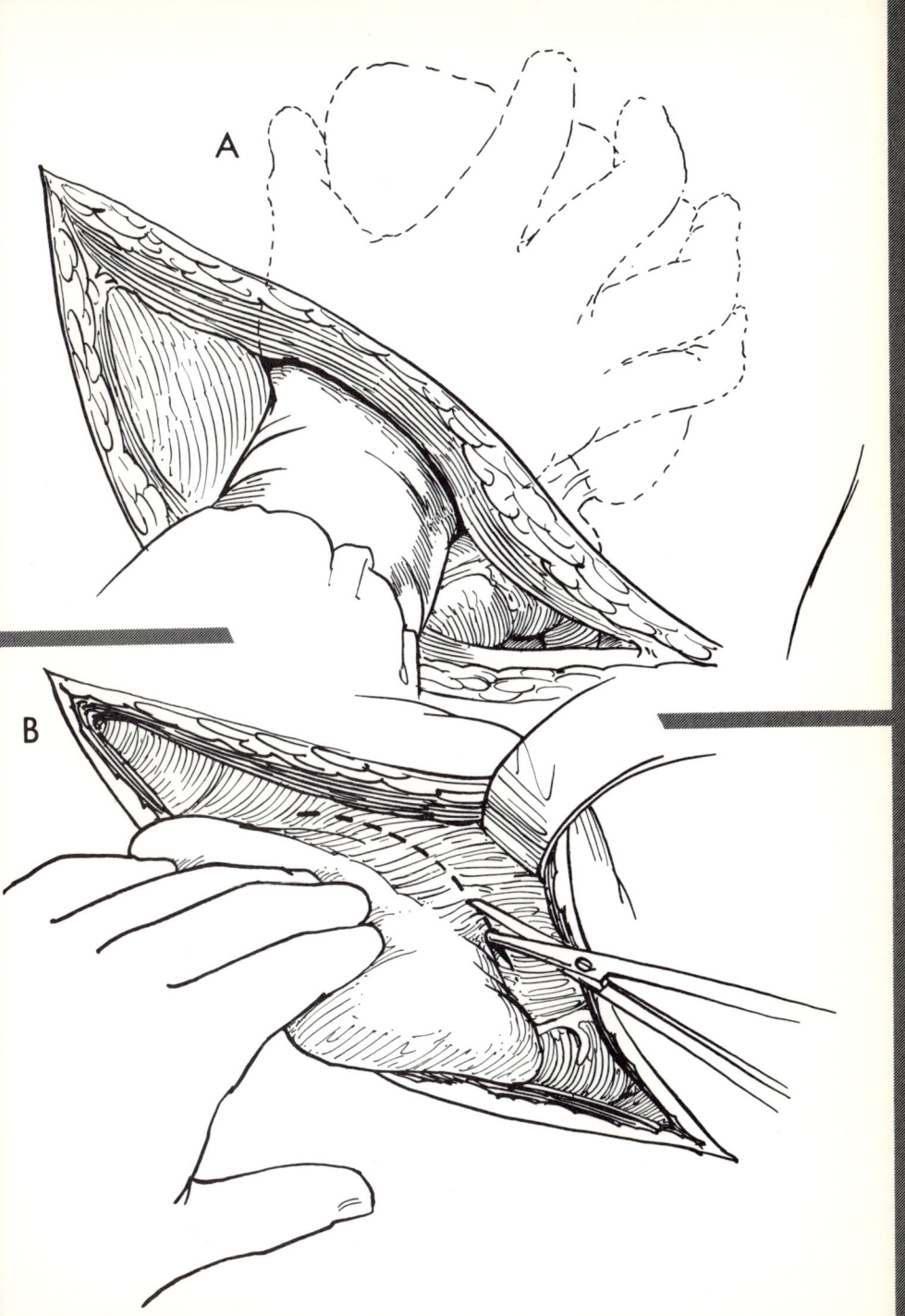

With blunt and sharp dissection, hemostasis being assured at every step, the spleen, the tail of the pancreas, the splenic vessels and the body of the stomach are mobilized further **(C)** until the left border of the aorta is exposed. The spleen and the pancreatic tail are covered with a laparotomy pad and retracted medially. The renal fascia (Gerota's) is opened. The left adrenal is now well exposed.

The left adrenal vein is dissected, proximal to its trifurcation. The lateral and medial borders and caudal end of the gland are mobilized **(D)**. The surgeon grasps the gland with his left hand and applies gentle caudal traction to facilitate the exposure and dissection of the nerve bundles at the medial superior border.

Again the gland is delivered intact, with a generous layer of periadrenal fat. Complete hemostasis is ascertained. There is no need or indication for drains.

[Approach by reflection of the spleen *continued on page 242.*]

PLATE 46

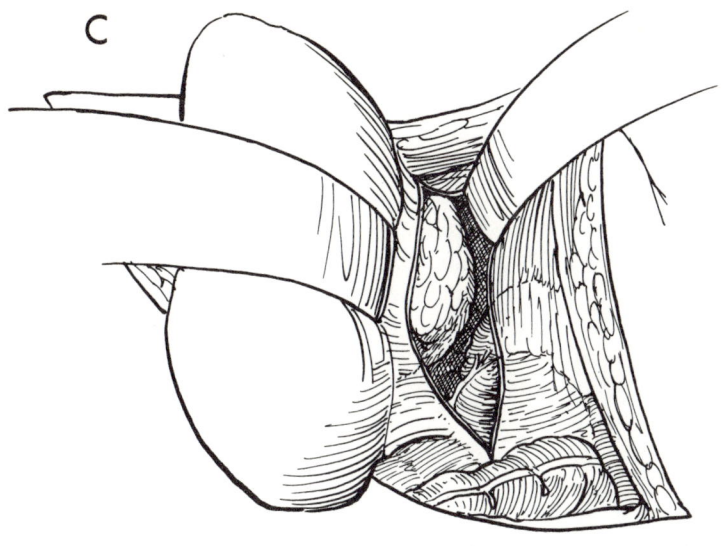

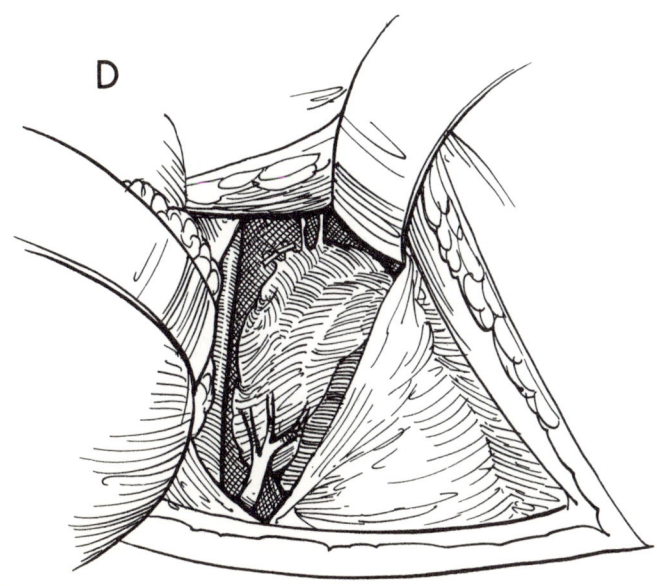

Adrenalectomy: Abdominal Transperitoneal Approach

The approach to the left adrenal gland by reflection of the spleen is understood best by the study of the anatomy of the abdomen and peritoneal reflections as seen in cross-sections. In the first 2 sketches **(E** and **F)** the reader is standing at the feet of the subject and looks at the cross-section of the upper half of the body, transected at the level of the 2 kidneys. The interrupted arrow in the first sketch delineates the course of the dissection around the lateral border of the spleen, through the splenorenal ligament and into the retroperitoneal space, posterior to the pancreas and anterior to the aorta, left kidney and adrenal **(E)**. The degree of dissection that this approach entails is minimal. Great care must be taken to avoid tears of the splenic capsule, especially near the site of ligamentous attachments.

Closure

Once the procedure is completed, the incision is closed in 2 fascial layers for the transverse (subcostal) incision and 1 fascial layer for the midline incisions. Sutures in the subcutaneous space are of little value; they produce devitalization of the fat layer and set the stage for wound infection. If there is a large subcutaneous dead space, this is eliminated best by plastic catheter suction.

The skin is approximated by a few interrupted 5-0 sutures and $\frac{1}{2}$-in adhesive tapes **(G)**. A light dressing is applied.

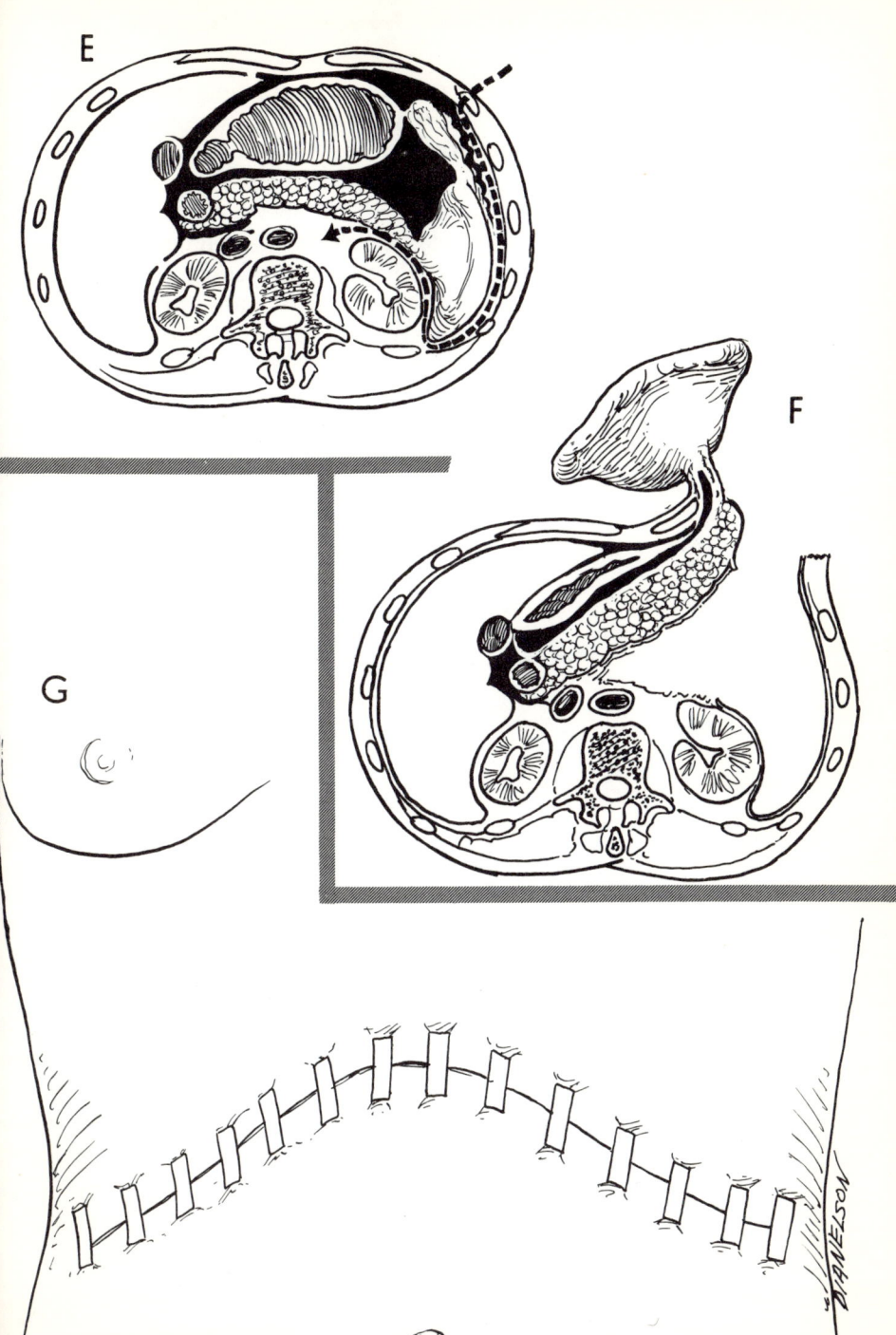

ELEVATION OF PANCREAS FOR EXPOSURE OF LEFT ADRENAL. — Theoretically this is the most direct approach to the left adrenal and requires a minimal amount of dissection.

The gastrocolic ligament is exposed; dissection begins in the avascular segment, toward the left, until the lesser peritoneal cavity is entered (A). The surgeon holds the index and middle fingers of his left hand in the opening to facilitate further dissection by elevating the gastrocolic ligament. Dissection of this ligament proceeds until it is divided from the gastric antrum to the level of the short gastric vessels (B). Division of a few of the short gastrics may be advisable in some instances.

The tail and body of the pancreas are now well exposed (C). The interrupted line at the inferior border of the tail of the pancreas delineates the next line of the dissection; it should be at least 1 cm removed from the pancreatic border to avoid injury to the pancreas and to provide adequate pedicles for the vessels that require ligation. The body of the stomach is retracted rostrally, with a Harrington or with a Spring retractor.

[Elevation of pancreas for exposure of left adrenal *continued on page 246*.]

PLATE 47

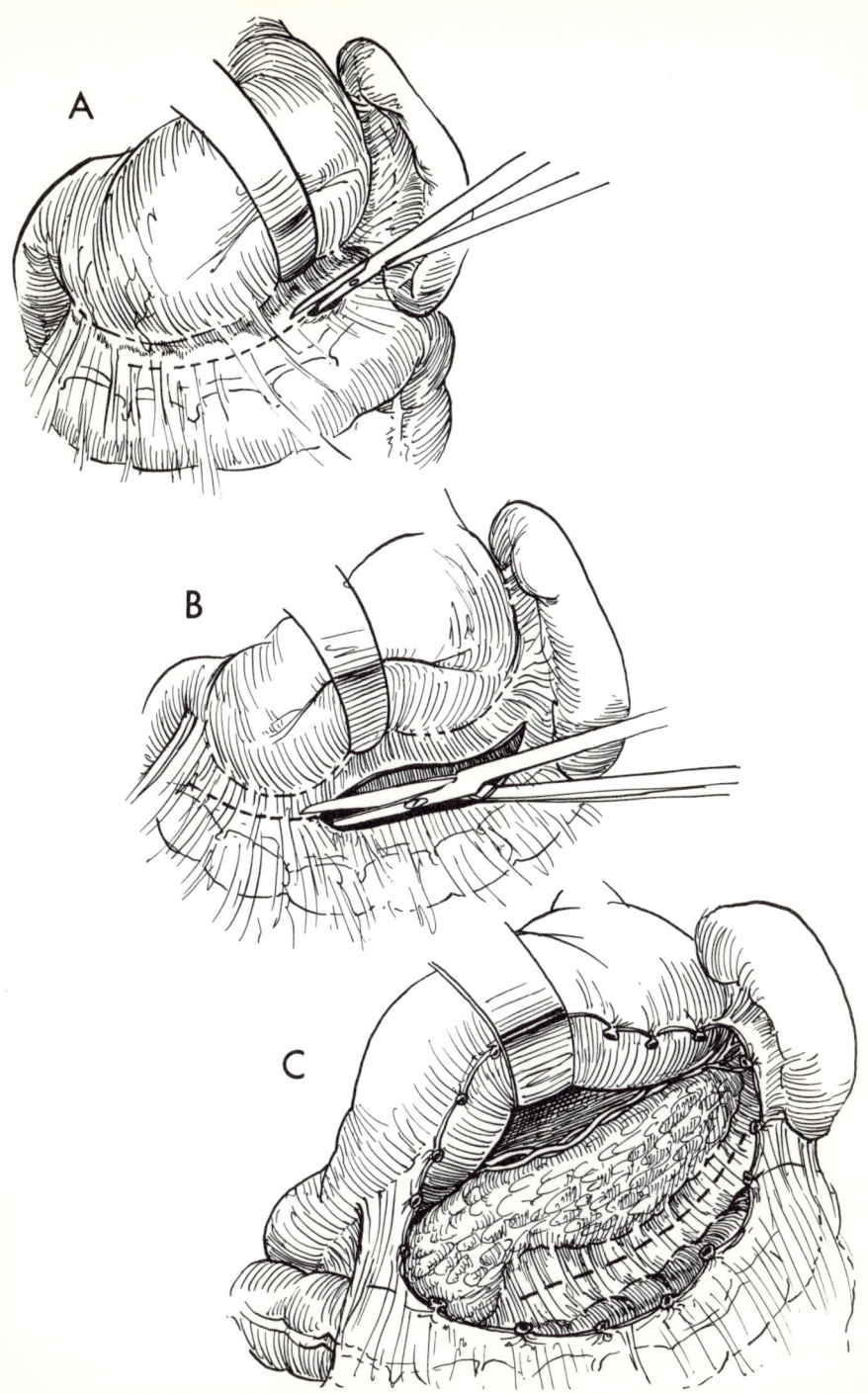

The posterior parietal peritoneum of the lesser peritoneal cavity is divided along the inferior border of the tail and body of the pancreas, along a line approximately 1 cm removed from it **(D)**. With gentle blunt dissection, the posterior retroperitoneal surface of the pancreas is dissected. During this dissection the inferior mesenteric vein is encountered, entering the splenic vein near the junction of the third and fourth portion of the duodenum. (These structures have been omitted from the sketches for the sake of simplicity.)

The tail and body of the pancreas can be elevated very gently with a Harrington or a Spring retractor (with blunt edges). Separate retraction of the body of the stomach is no longer required. The pararenal fat is dissected and perirenal fat layer is entered by opening the renal (Gerota's) fascia.

The left adrenal gland is visualized **(E)**. The adrenal vein is dissected, ligated and divided just proximal to its trifurcation. Dissection of the gland proceeds according to the method described in the previous (Reflection of the Spleen) section.

Hemostasis is ascertained. The pancreas is allowed to return to its anatomic position. There is no need to close the large defect in the gastrocolic ligament, provided the greater omentum is draped over the small bowel. In the absence of greater omentum, the defect should be closed to obviate the possibility of internal herniation. There is no necessity for drainage.

THORACOABDOMINAL INCISION

The indication for a thoracoabdominal incision is the presence of an unusually large adrenal tumor. The possibility of a malignancy invading adjacent structures must then be considered and adequate exposure for en bloc resection provided.

In such a situation an abdominal incision is still preferable to a flank approach for 2 reasons: (1) both adrenal fossas can be explored through a single incision; (2) better visualization and control of major vessels is obtained.

A transverse upper abdominal incision is made first. The abdomen is explored. The incision is extended into the seventh or eighth interspace on the appropriate side. The ensuing procedure depends on the particular situation. Malignancies should be resected in the classic manner, with an adequate margin of normal tissue.

PLATE 47

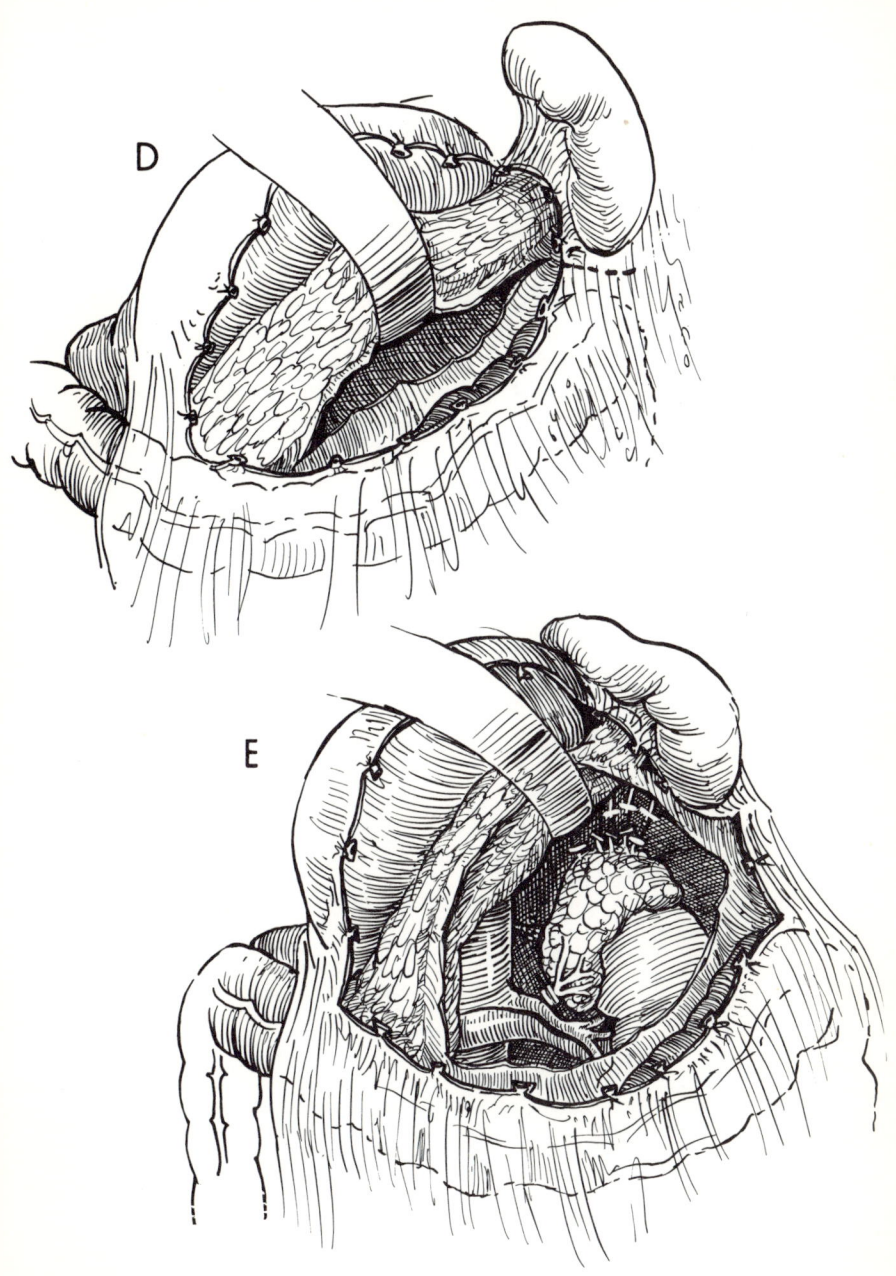

Posterior Thoracolumbar Approach

ANATOMIC CONSIDERATIONS. — These are illustrated in Plate 48.

The right adrenal and kidney are situated more caudally than their counterparts on the left. Since a substantial portion of the right adrenal is retrocaval, the posterior approach simplifies the dissection of this gland and the identification and ligation of its vein(s).

Greater traction must be exerted on the left kidney (as compared to the right) to bring the left adrenal into the field of dissection, after resection of the twelfth rib.

The tail of the pancreas can be mistaken for the left adrenal. This mistake can be obviated by good hemostasis and good illumination, which should allow the surgeon to discern between the pinkish white pancreas and the orange-colored adrenal.

One of the great advantages of the thoracolumbar approach is that these incisions produce minimal wound pain; this allows rapid ambulation of the patient.

Since the entire dissection, bilaterally, is extraperitoneal, postoperative ileus is minimal and is due solely to edema of the retroperitoneal autonomic nerve plexuses.

[Posterior thoracolumbar approach *continued on page 250.*]

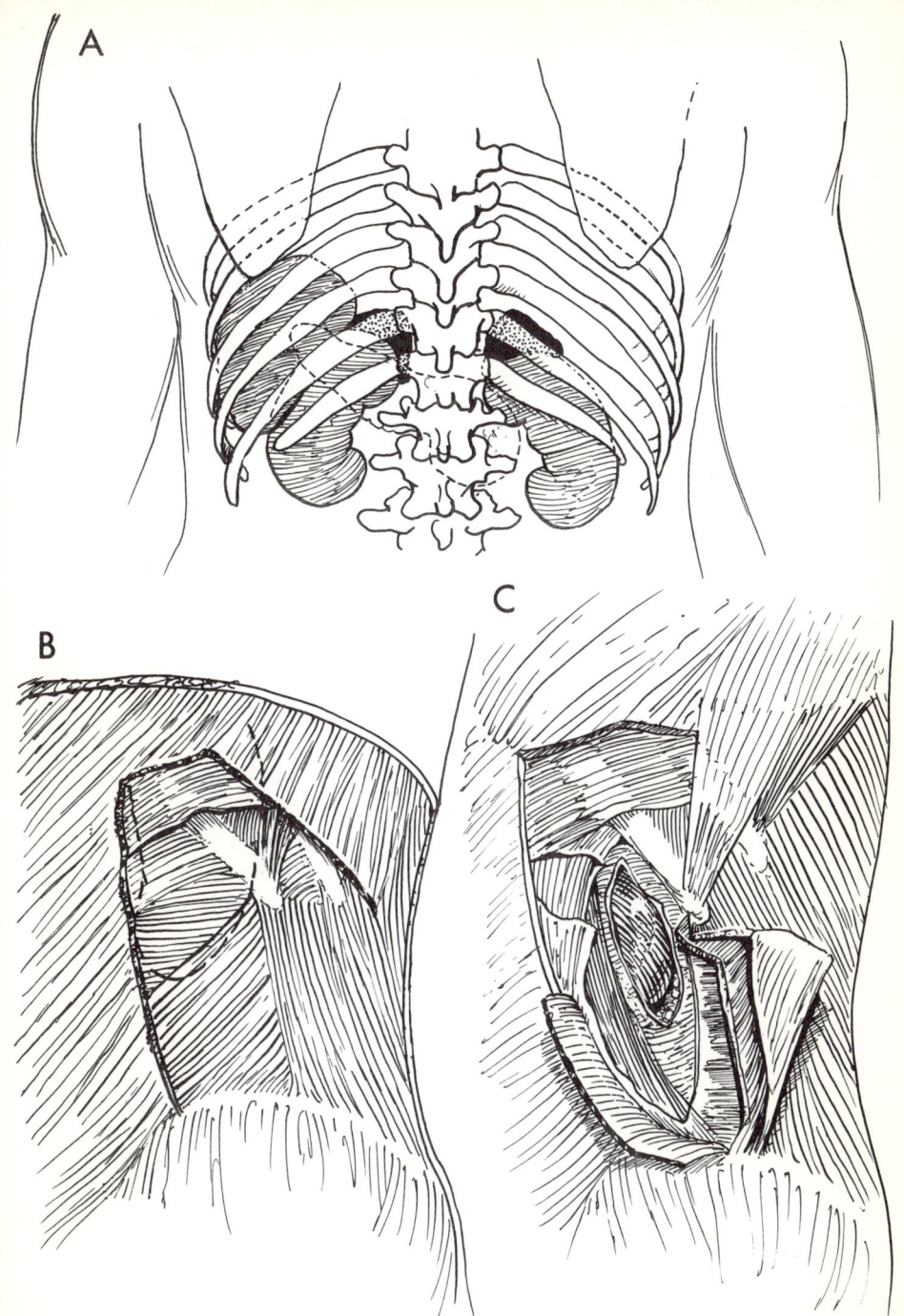

Adrenalectomy: Posterior Thoracolumbar Approach

POSITIONING OF THE PATIENT. — After the endotracheal tube is in place and well secured, the patient is turned into the prone position. To assure adequate ventilation, 2 foam-rubber blocks (inset) are placed longitudinally under the shoulders and the lateral aspect of the thorax down to the pelvis **(D)**. It is important to assure adequate support under the shoulders to avoid excessive pressure and traction on the brachial plexus. A foam-rubber doughnut is placed under the head.

The umbilicus of the patient is aligned with the break in the table. The table is angulated to flex the patient's body at the hip joints to the point where the skin overlying the twelfth rib is taut. This widens the distance between the intercostal spaces and between the costal margin and the iliac crest. Furthermore, along with the abdominal pressure provided by the foam-rubber blocks, this maneuver brings the kidneys and adrenals in a position closer to the back of the patient, and thus facilitates their exposure and dissection.

The entire operating table is adjusted at this point to place the thorax and lumbodorsal surface of the patient in a horizontal position, parallel to the floor. The table should be flexed at the knees to minimize venous stasis; the legs may be wrapped with Ace bandages or elastic stockings for the same purpose.

The importance of accurate positioning of the patient cannot be overemphasized.

INCISIONS. — The incisions are slightly oblique. The left incision is approximately 1.5 cm rostral to the right **(E)**. The relationship of the ribs to the incisions and to the pleural reflection on the right is indicated in **F**.

[Posterior thoracolumbar approach *continued on page 252.*]

PLATE 48

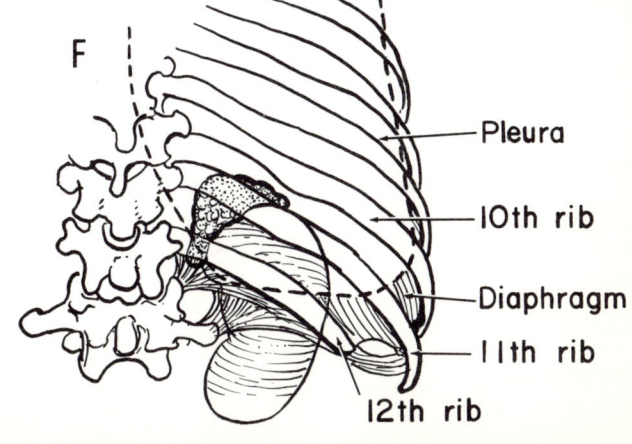

D

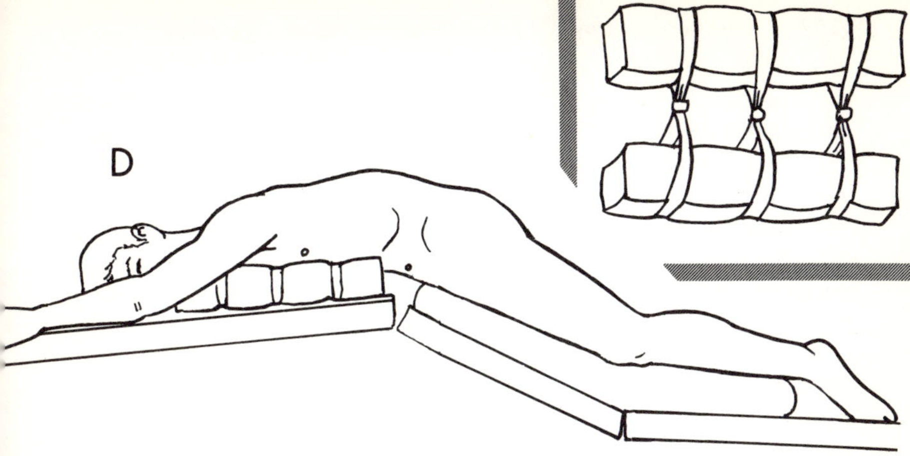

E

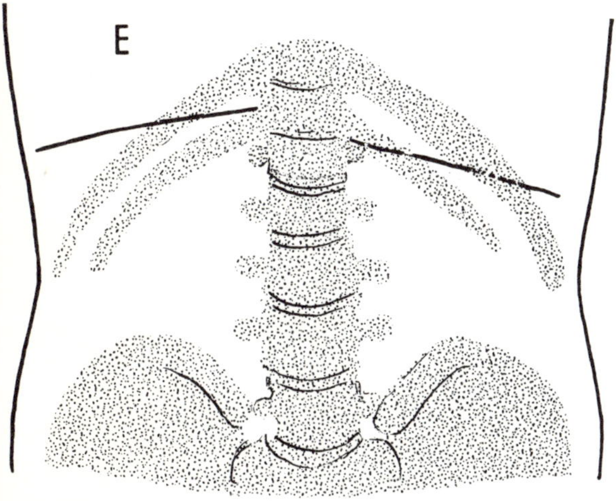

F
- Pleura
- 10th rib
- Diaphragm
- 11th rib
- 12th rib

The skin incisions extend from the vertebral border to the lateral costal margin. The incision continues **(G)** through subcutaneous fat, the latissimus dorsi, the posterior inferior serratus and the periosteum of the twelfth rib.

The periosteum of the twelfth rib is incised along the midline of the rib. Periosteal elevators and a Doyen rib elevator are used to mobilize the rib from a lateral to a medial direction **(H and I)**.

The fascia covering the sacrospinal muscle is incised longitudinally, to allow medial retraction of this muscle with a Brewster retractor and to expose the medial end of the twelfth rib.

The lateral end of the twelfth rib is detached from the external and internal oblique and transversus abdominis muscles with heavy scissors. The rib is resected.

[Posterior thoracolumbar approach *continued on page 254.*]

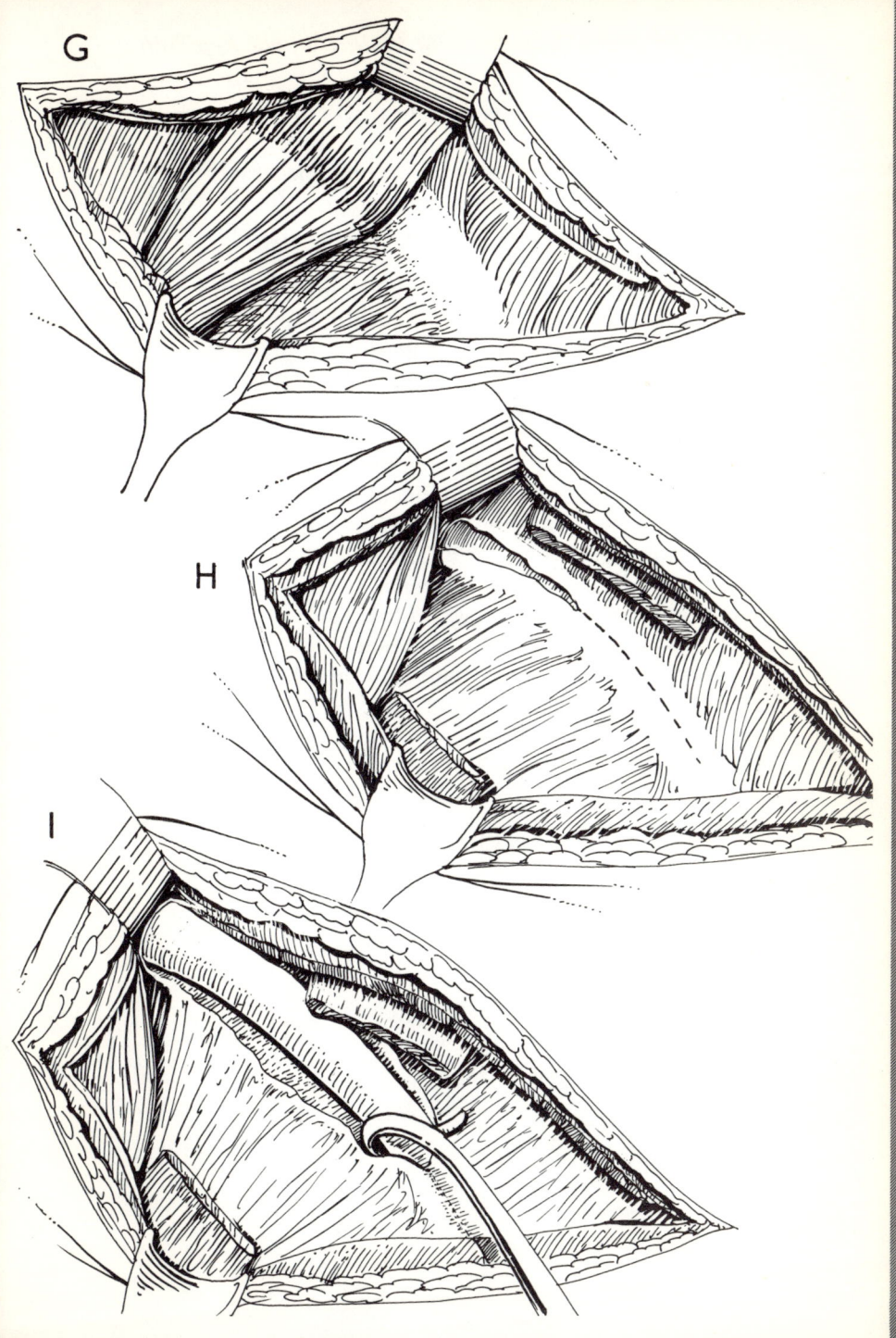

Adrenalectomy: Posterior Thoracolumbar Approach

A box-type rib cutter is used to resect an additional 2–3 cm of rib medially **(J)**.

Resection of the eleventh rib is seldom necessary.

During the resection of the tip of the twelfth rib from its attachments to the external and internal oblique and transversus abdominis muscles, the lumbodorsal (transversalis) fascia is usually penetrated. This opening is then extended medially and laterally **(K)**. Great care is taken not to enter the pleural space. After the twelfth rib has been resected, the pleuroperitoneal demarcation is usually clearly evident along a line which runs almost transversely and crosses the bed of the twelfth rib near the costovertebral angle (see Plate 48, **E** and **F**).

Once the paranephric retroperitoneal fat is dissected, a transverse incision is made in the perinephric (Gerota's) fascia **(L)**. This permits caudal retraction of the kidney with a large Harrington retractor. This maneuver moves the adrenal gland caudally into plain view. Occasionally the right adrenal gland is fixed in position and somewhat removed and detached from the superomedial aspect of the kidney; when the kidney is retracted caudally, the right adrenal may then remain in its original position **(M)**. A certain degree of dexterity and excellent lighting may be required to localize and resect it. In such instances the vena cava is first located and dissected gently in a rostral direction, until the right adrenal is encountered.

[Posterior thoracolumbar approach *continued on page 256.*]

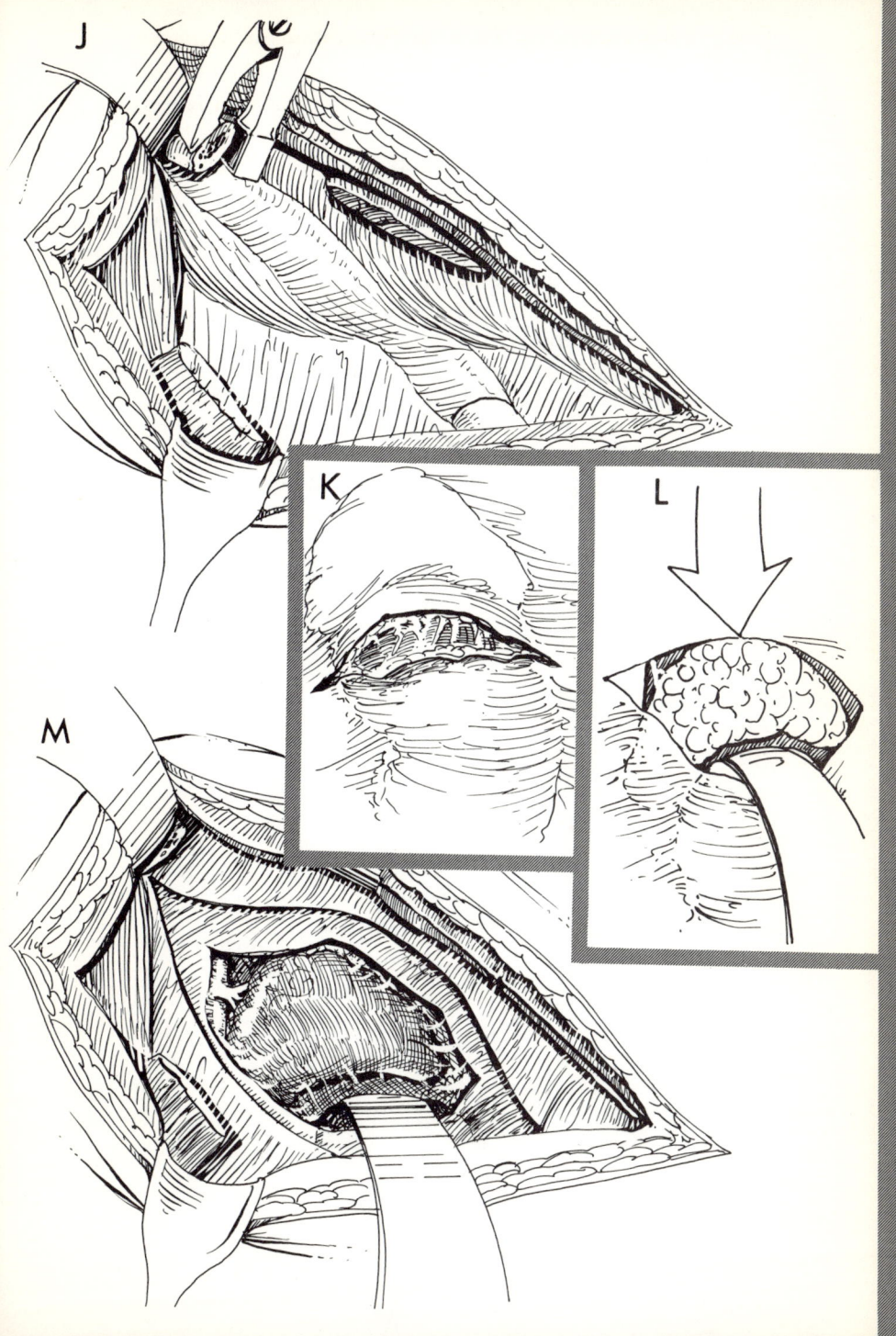

Once the adrenal gland is exposed **(N)** the vein is located, dissected, doubly clipped and divided.

The lateral and inferior aspects of the gland are dissected with great care to assure hemostasis.

The nerve bundles at the superomedial aspect of the gland are the last structures to be divided between clips **(O)**. Once the entire gland is dissected sufficiently, caudal and lateral traction may be achieved to expose and dissect these nerve bundles, which are otherwise difficult to reach.

The right adrenal gland may be adherent to the liver. In such an instance great care should be exerted to avoid injury to the liver and leakage of bile. If there is any question, the wound must be drained.

Vigorous dissection of the right adrenal may tear the vena cava, especially if the adrenal gland or the tumor is firmly adherent.

[Closure *on page 258*.]

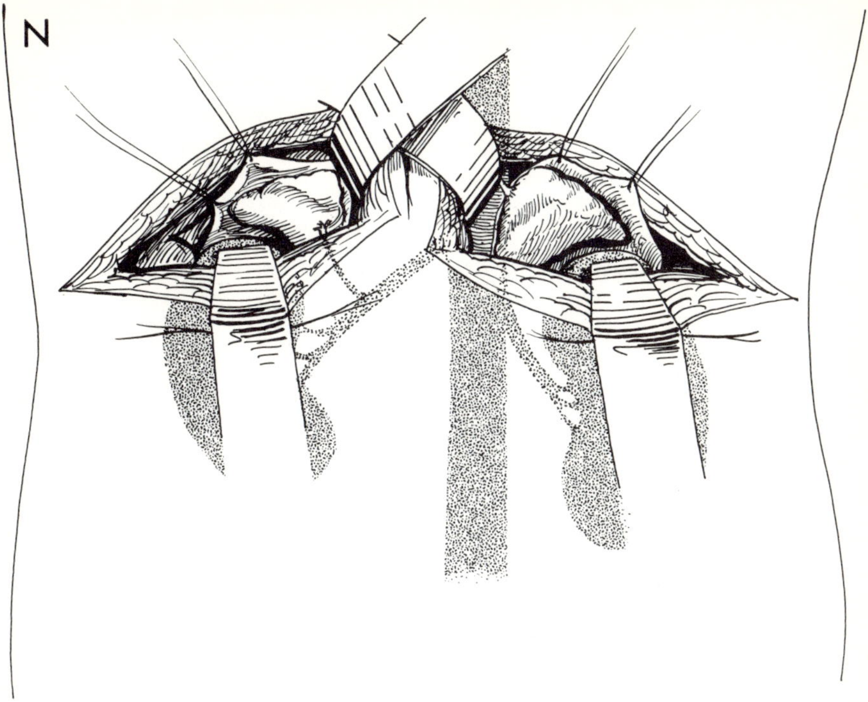

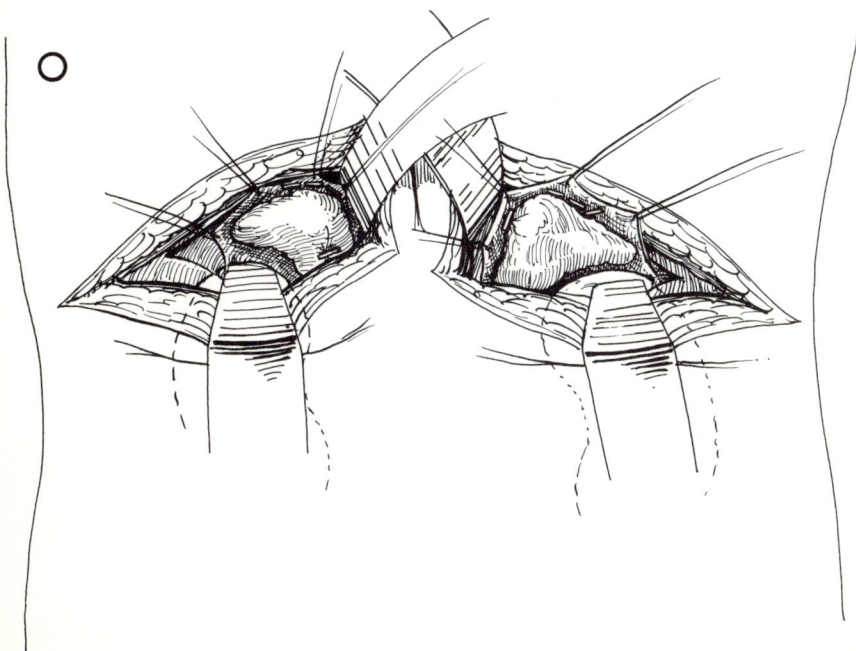

CLOSURE. — Once the gland is removed, the incision is closed in layers. All fascial layers except the perirenal fascia are closed (**P** and **Q**). Drainage is not necessary unless injury to the pancreas or the liver is suspected. The subcutaneous tissues do not require sutures. The skin is closed with interrupted nylon or wire, since these sutures must remain for 3 weeks (**R**).

FLANK APPROACH

In rare instances of unilateral massive adrenal tumors, where malignancy is very likely and en bloc resection with surrounding tissue is indicated, the flank approach provides superb exposure, especially on the right side.

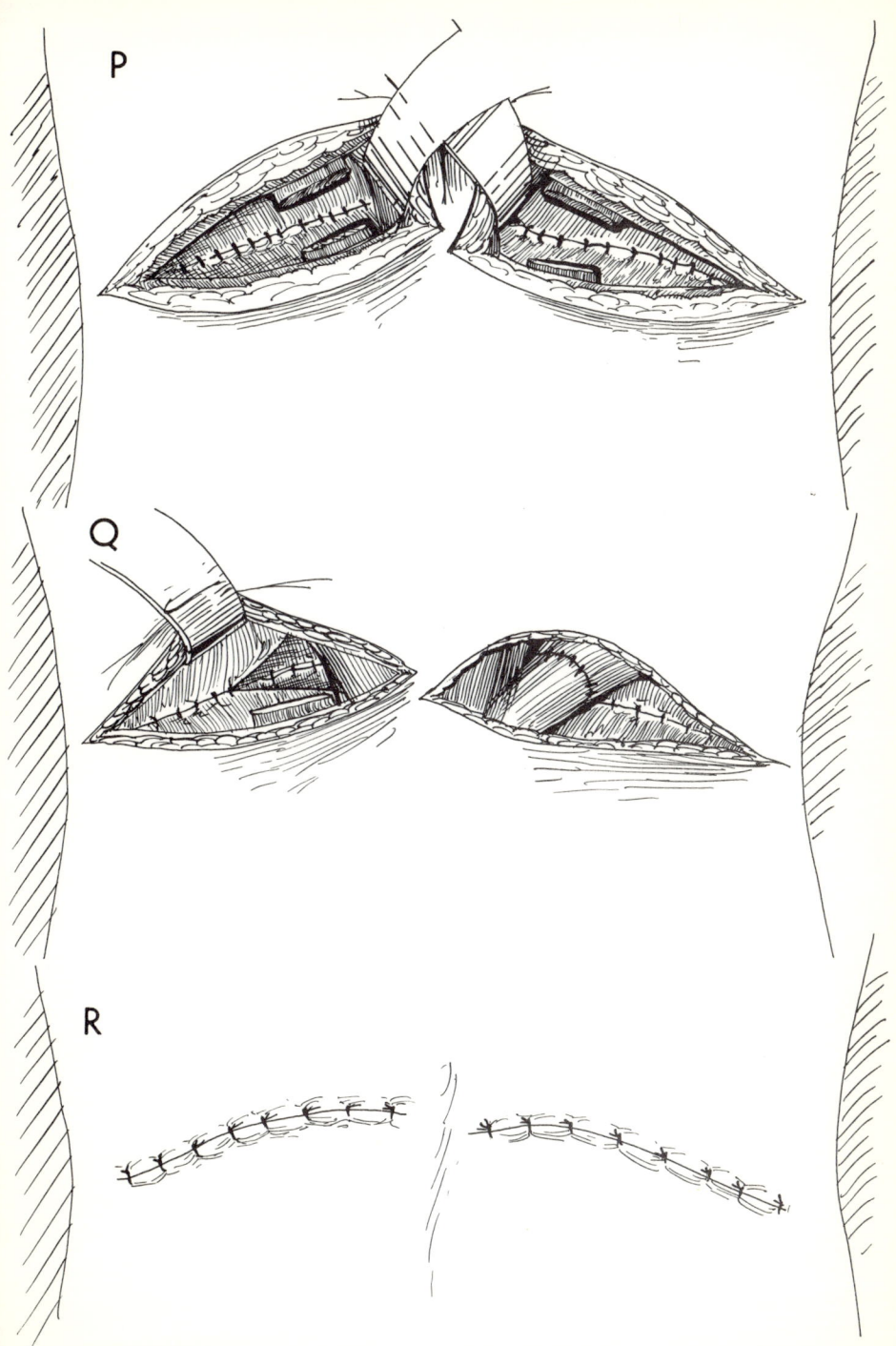

CHAPTER 5

The Future of Endocrine Surgery

The great strides achieved in endocrinology during the past 20 years are amazing. With the application of modern technologic developments, our understanding of endocrinopathies has progressed to the point where endocrine diseases are diagnosed many years before they develop the full-blown clinical picture described in textbooks of recent vintage. Diabetes is diagnosed in the incipient stages of reactive hypoglycemia! Medullary carcinomas of the thyroid and pheochromocytomas are detected at the hyperplasia stage in young children of parents with the fully developed disease by means of provocative tests and exquisitely sensitive assays!

These advances have created a new set of problems for the clinician. How can one be certain that the children of a patient with Sipple's syndrome who have C cell hyperplasia of the thyroid gland and adrenal medullary hyperplasia will eventually develop carcinomas? Is total thyroidectomy or bilateral adrenalectomy justified at such a stage of the disease? Does the chain of events that begins as hyperplasia always eventuate into a metastatic carcinoma?

With the advent of successful autotransplantation of endocrine tissue, the surgeon may not be so reluctant to perform a bilateral adrenalectomy if he can successfully transplant functioning adrenal cortical tissue in an accessible site in case resection is required at a future date.

It is a fair assumption that many, if not most, endocrine tumors may be genetically predetermined; they will continue to be recognized in greater numbers, and many of them will require operative correction.

The role of endocrine surgeons will depend upon their level of interest, their sophistication in endocrinology and finally their willingness to translate these rapid developments into refinements that will reduce operative morbidity and enhance surgical cures, and to continue to capitalize on their unique position in developing new insights into the pathogenesis and treatment of endocrine disease.

From this vantage point the authors believe that endocrine surgery is both challenging and intellectually rewarding.

Index

A

Abdominal transperitoneal approach
  (see Adrenalectomy, abdominal
  transperitoneal approach)
Adenoma: toxic, 87, 93
Adrenal(s), 206–259
  anatomy of, 210–211
  diagnosis of surgically managed
    diseases, 212–233
  embryology of, 208–210
  histology of, 210–211
  pathophysiology of surgically
    managed diseases, 212–233
  secretion control, and
    steroidogenesis, 207–208
  surgical approaches to, 234–258
    in adrenalectomy (see under
      Adrenalectomy)
    anatomic considerations in,
      234–235
  tumors, masculinizing, feminizing and
    nonfunctioning 222
    causes of, 222
    clinical features of, 222
    diagnosis of, 222
    treatment of, 222
Adrenalectomy, 236–258
  abdominal transperitoneal approach
    to adrenal
    left, 238–239
    right, 236–237
  closure of, 242–243, 258
  flank approach, 258–259
  pancreas elevation to expose left
    adrenal, 244–246
  posterior thoracolumbar approach to,
    248–258
    anatomic considerations in,
      248–249
    closure of, 258

  incisions, 250–257
  positioning patient for, 250–251
  reflection of spleen approach,
    238–242
  thoracoabdominal incision in,
    246–247
Adrenergic stimulation: effects of, 229
Air embolism: and thyroid surgery,
  120–121
Airway
  obstruction, and thyroid surgery, 121
  problems, after parathyroidectomy,
    57
Aldosteronism, 218–221
  causes of, 218
  clinical manifestations of, 219
Amine-producing tumors, 223–233
Anabolic steroids, 22
Androgens, 22
Anesthesia: for parathyroidectomy,
  49–50
Anomalies: thyroglossal duct, 92
Aspiration cytology: of thyroid tumors,
  92
Autotransplantation: of parathyroid, 63

B

Beta cell tumors, 184–185
  diazoxide for, 184–185
  metastatic, and streptozotocin, 185
Biopsy: of islet cell tumors, 154–155
Bleeding (see Hemorrhage)
Bone signs: of hyperparathyroidism,
  42–43

C

Calcareous disease: renal, and
  hyperparathyroidism, 36–37, 77
Calcitonin, 22

Calcium
  homeostasis, regulation of, 20-22
  infusion, IV, in gastrinoma diagnosis, 188-189
  salt deposition in kidney after parathyroidectomy, 58
Cancer
  pheochromocytoma, malignant, 233
  thyroid, 89, 93-94
    medullary, 227
    medullary, and pheochromocytoma, 233
  after surgery, 125
Carcinoma: of parathyroid, 72-73
Catecholamines
  degradation of, 228
  synthesis of, 228
Cell (*see* Beta cell tumors)
Chemistries: abnormal, in hyperparathyroidism, 40-41
Children: pheochromocytoma of, 233
Cholera, pancreatic (*see* Islet cell tumors, diarrheogenic)
Chromaffin tumors: embryologic derivation of, 226
Coma: and acute hypercalcemia, 72
Complications (*see* Thyroid, complications of surgery)
Corneal abrasion: and thyroid surgery, 123
Cushing's syndrome, 212-218
  causes of, 212
  clinical manifestations of, 213
  diagnosis of, 213-215
    differential, 214-215
  surgery of, intraoperative management and surprises, 217-218
  treatment of, 216-218
Cyst: thyroglossal duct, excision of, 118-119
Cytology: aspiration, of thyroid tumors, 92

D

Diarrheogenic islet cell tumors (*see* Islet cell tumors, diarrheogenic)
Diazoxide
  for beta cell tumors, 184-185
  suppression test, in insulinoma, 159
Drains: after thyroidectomy, 98-99

E

Embolism: air, and thyroid surgery, 120-121
Embryologic derivation: of chromaffin tumors, 226
Embryology
  of adrenals, 208-210
  of pancreas, 138-139
  of thyroid, 80-81
Endocrine
  surgery, future of, 260-261
  tumors, multiple, and primary hyperparathyroidism, 44
Enucleation of tumors
  islet cell, ectopic, 178-182
    closure after, 182-183
  pancreatic head, 172-176
Esophagojejunostomy, 196-201
Estrogens, 22
Extrapancreatic neoplasms, 185

F

Feminizing tumors (*see* Adrenal, tumors, masculinizing, feminizing)
Flank approach: in adrenalectomy, 258-259
Flap: skin, development of, and parathyroidectomy, 50-52
Future: of endocrine surgery, 260-261

G

Ganglioneuroma, 226
Gastrectomy: total, for gastrinoma, 190-203
Gastrin, 131
  circulating, in gastrinoma diagnosis, 188
Gastrinoma, 186-203
  clinical manifestations of, 186-187
  diagnosis of, 188-189
    differential, 189
  gastrectomy for, total, 190-203
  history of, 186
  radiography of, 189
Gastrocolic ligament division: to expose pancreas, 148-151
Glucagon, 22, 130-131
Glucagonoma, 205

Goiter
  diffuse, nontoxic, 88
  multinodular, 88
  toxic, 86-87
Gout: and hyperparathyroidism, 77
Graves' disease, 86, 93
  resection for, bilateral subtotal, 114

H

Hemorrhage
  after parathyroidectomy, 58
  in thyroid surgery, 120
  postoperative, 122
History
  of gastrinoma, 186
  of islet cell tumors, 129
    diarrheogenic, 204
  of pancreas (*see* Pancreas, history of)
Homeostasis of calcium: regulation of, 20-22
Hormone, parathyroid, 20
  excess, effects of, 39
Hyperaldosteronism, 218-221
  clinical manifestations of, 219
  primary
    diagnosis of, 219-221
    diagnosis of, differential, 220-221
    surgery of, unusual intraoperative problems, 221-222
    treatment of, 221
Hypercalcemia
  acute, and coma, 72
  diagnosis of, differential, 22-23
  effects of, 39
  pancreatic mass and, 75
  rebound after acute pancreatitis, 74
Hyperparathyroidism
  bone signs of, 42-43
  diagnosis, and parathyroidectomy, 47-49
  history of, milestones, by year, 19
  hyperthyroidism coexisting with, 74
  joint signs of, 42-43
  primary, 34-41
    abnormal chemistries in, 40-41
    clinical forms of, 34-35
    disorders associated with, 44-46
    renal calcareous disease and, 36-37, 77
    signs of, 38-39
    symptoms of, 38-39

  renal, 68-71
    diagnosis of, 69
    parathyroidectomy in (*see* Parathyroidectomy, in renal hyperparathyroidism)
    pathology of, 68
  secondary (*see* renal *above*)
  thyroid tumors coexisting with, 44-46, 73
Hypertension: and primary hyperparathyroidism, 44, 76
Hyperthyroidism: coexisting with hyperparathyroidism, 84
Hypocalcemia
  after parathyroidectomy, management of, 60-62
  after thyroid surgery, 122-123
Hypoglycemia, 156-157
  clinical manifestations of, 156
  diagnosis of, differential, 156-157
  fasting, in insulinoma, 158
Hypokalemia: differential diagnosis of, 221

I

Instruments: for parathyroidectomy, 50
Insulin, 130
Insulinoma, 158-163
  diagnosis of, 158-161
  diazoxide suppression test in, 159
  hypoglycemia in, fasting, 158
  postoperative management, 184
  provocative tests in, 159
  radiographic localization, 160-161
  treatment, 162-163
Islet cell tumors, 126-205
  biopsy of, 154-155
  classification of, 134
  diarrheogenic, 204-205
    clinical features of, 204
    diagnosis, 204-205
    history of, 204
    treatment, 205
  ectopic, 178-183
    enucleation of, 178-181
    enucleation of, closure after, 182-183
  histopathology of, 136-138
  history of, 129
  location of, 134-136
  size of, 134-136

Index

Islets of pancreas, 127–128
  histology of, 131–133
  physiology of, 130–131

J

Jejunojejunostomy, 201–202
Joint signs: of hyperparathyroidism, 42–43

K

Keloids: after thyroid surgery, 124
Kidney
  calcareous disease, and hyperparathyroidism, 36–37, 77
  calcium salt deposition in, after parathyroidectomy, 58
  hyperparathyroidism (see Hyperparathyroidism, renal)

L

Laryngeal nerve palsy: after thyroid surgery, 124
Ligament: gastrocolic, division to expose pancreas, 148–151
Lobectomy: thyroid, 100–101

M

Malignancy (see Cancer)
Masculinizing tumors (see Adrenal[s], tumors, masculinizing)
Metabolic histories of pancreas, 127–129
Metastatic beta cell tumors: and streptozotocin, 185
Microscopy: of parathyroid, 26–27

N

Neck dissection: in total thyroidectomy, 104–113
Neoplasms (see Tumors)
Nerve
  laryngeal, palsy after thyroid surgery, 124
  recurrent
    palsy, after thyroid surgery, 123–124
    severed, and thyroidectomy, 121
Neuroblastoma, 226

P

Pancreas, 126–205
  anatomy of, 140–143
  cholera (see Islet cell tumors, diarrheogenic)
  elevation to expose left adrenal, 244–246
  embryology of, 138–139
  examination of head and uncinate process, 152–153
  exposure of
    body, 148–151
    by division of gastrocolic ligament, 148–151
    head, 152–153
    tail, 148–151
    uncinate process, 152–153
  history of
    highlights of, 126–129
    metabolic, 127–129
    morphologic, 126–127
  islet cell tumors of (see Islet cell tumors)
  islets of (see Islets of pancreas)
  mass, and hypercalcemia, 75
  metabolism of, 127–129
  morphology, 126–127
  surgical approaches to, 144–147
  tumors, 164–177
  tumors, in body, 164–173
    resection of, 164–169
    resection of, closure after, 170–171
  tumors, extrapancreatic, 185
  tumors, in head, 172–176
    enucleation, 172–176
    enucleation on posterior surface, 176
  tumors, in tail, 164–173
    resection of, 164–169
    resection of, closure after, 170–171
  tumors, within uncinate process, 176–177
Pancreatitis
  acute
    after parathyroidectomy, 58
    rebound hypercalcemia after, 74
  chronic, and primary hyperparathyroidism, 46
Parathyroid, 18–77
  anatomy of, 24–27

Index [267]

developmental, 24–25
autotransplantation, 63
carcinoma, 72–73
enlarged, location of, 32–33
function, normal, 20–21
gross appearance of, 26–27
historical perspective on, 18–19
hormone, 20
  excess, effects of, 39
identification of, 52–53
inferior, location of, 30–31
microscopic appearance of, 26–27
pathology of, 59–60
reimplantation, and thyroidectomy, 121
superior, location of, 28–29
tissue excision extent for parathyroidectomy, 54
tumors, aberrant or overlooked at parathyroidectomy, localization of, 64–66
Parathyroidectomy, 47–67
  aberrant tumors after, localization of, 64–66
  airway problems after, 57
  anesthesia for, 49–50
  calcium salt deposition in kidney after, 58
  closure, 54
  follow-up after, long-term, 62–63
  hemorrhage after, 58
  hyperparathyroidism diagnosis and, 47–49
  hypocalcemia after, management of, 60–62
  incision for, 50–52
  indications for, 47–49
  instruments for, 50
  overlooked tumors, localization of, 64–66
  pancreatitis after, acute, 58
  parenchyma in, 54
  positioning for, 50
  postoperative care, 56–59
    in first 24 hours, 56–58
    routine, 56–59
    in second 24 hours, 59
  re-exploration after, 63–67
  operative technic, 66–67
  in renal hyperparathyroidism, 69–71
    diagnosis and, 69
    discussion of, 70–71

follow-up of, long-term, 71
indications for, 69
results of, 71
results of, 59, 71
skin flap development and, 50–52
thyroid mobilization and, 52–53
tissue excision in, extent of, 54
Parenchyma: in parathyroidectomy, 54
Peptic ulcer: and primary hyperparathyroidism, 46, 77
Pheochromocytoma, 223–233
  bilateral, 232
  causes of, 223–225
  in children, 233
  clinical features of, 227–228
  diagnosis of, 228–230
  malignant, 233
  postoperative management in, 232
  during pregnancy, 232
  thyroid cancer and, medullary, 233
  treatment of, 230–232
Plummer's disease, 86–87
Postoperative
  complications of thyroid surgery, 121–124
  management
    of insulinoma, 184
    after parathyroidectomy (see Parathyroidectomy, postoperative care)
    in pheochromocytoma, 232
    after thyroid surgery, 125
Pregnancy: pheochromocytoma during, 232
Preoperative management: in thyroidectomy, 94
Provocative tests: in insulinoma, 159
Pseudogout: and primary hyperparathyroidism, 46, 77
Pseudohyperparathyroidism, 75–76
PTH, 20
  excess, effects of, 39

R

Radiography
  of gastrinoma, 189
  of insulinoma, 160–161
Reimplantation: of parathyroid, and thyroidectomy, 121
Renal (see Kidney)

Index

S

Scar: asymmetric, after thyroid surgery, 124
Skin flap development: and parathyroidectomy, 50-52
Spleen: reflection of spleen approach in adrenalectomy, 238-242
Steroidogenesis: and adrenal secretion control, 207-208
Steroids: anabolic, 22
Storm: thyroid, after surgery, 122
Streptozotocin: and metastatic beta cell tumors, 185

T

Thoracoabdominal incision: in adrenalectomy, 246-247
Thoracolumbar approach (see Adrenalectomy, posterior thoracolumbar approach)
Thyroglossal duct
  anomalies, 92
  cyst excision, 118-119
Thyroid, 78-125
  anatomy of, surgical, 80-81, 84-85
  cancer (see Cancer, thyroid)
  complications of surgery, 120-124
    intraoperative, 120-121
    postoperative, 121-124
  disease, benign, 93
  ectopic tissue, 82-83
  embryology of, 80-81
  exposure of, 94-95
  lingual, excision of, 120
  lobectomy, 100-101
  mobilization, and parathyroidectomy, 52-53
  nodule, excision of, 96-99
  pathophysiology from surgical viewpoint, 86-88
  storm, after surgery, 122
  tumors, 87-92
    benign, 89
    benign, after surgery, 125
    classification, 89
    clinical evaluation, 90-91
    cytology of, aspiration, 92
    histologic diagnosis short of surgery, 92

hyperparathyroidism coexisting with, 44-46, 73
Thyroidectomy
  air embolism and, 120-121
  airway obstruction and, 121
  bilateral subtotal, 114-117
  closure of, 98-99
  complications of (see Thyroid, complications of surgery)
  corneal abrasion after, 123
  drains after, 98-99
  excision of nodule, 96-99
  exposure of thyroid, 94-95
  hemorrhage after, 122
  hemorrhage during, 120
  hypocalcemia after, 122-123
  indications for, 93-94
  keloids after, 124
  nerve palsy after
    laryngeal, 124
    recurrent, 123-124
  parathyroid reimplantation and, 121
  postoperative management, 125
  preoperative management, 94
  scar after, asymmetric, 124
  severed nerve and, recurrent, 121
  thyroid storm after, 122
  thyrotoxic state after, 125
  total, 102-113
    with neck dissection, 104-113
  tumors after, benign and malignant, 125
Thyrotoxic state: after surgery, 125
Thyrotoxicosis, 86-87
Toxic
  adenoma, 87, 93
  goiter, multinodular, 86-87
Transplantation: of parathyroid, 63
Tumors
  adrenal (see Adrenal[s], tumors)
  amine-producing, 223-233
  beta cell (see Beta cell tumors)
  chromaffin, embryologic derivation of, 226
  endocrine, multiple, and primary hyperparathyroidism, 44
  feminizing (see Adrenal, tumors, masculinizing, feminizing)
  islet cell (see Islet cell tumors)
  malignant (see Cancer)
  masculinizing (see Adrenal, tumors,

masculinizing)
pancreas (*see* Pancreas, tumors)
parathyroid, aberrant or overlooked at parathyroidectomy, localization of, 64–66
thyroid (*see* Thyroid, tumors)

U

Ulcer: peptic, and primary hyperparathyroidism, 46, 77

V

Vitamin D, 20

W

WDHA syndrome (*see* Islet cell tumors, diarrheogenic)

X

X-ray (*see* Radiography)